Mood Disorders and Antidepressants

With the fully revised fourth edition of *Essential Psychopharmacology*, Dr Stahl returns to the essential roots of what it means to become a neurobiologically empowered psychopharmacologist, expertly guided in the selection and combination of treatments for individual patients in practice.

This remains the essential text for all students and professionals in mental health seeking to understand and utilize current therapeutics, and to anticipate the future for novel medications.

This special edition, featuring the extracted chapters on mood disorders and antidepressants, provides a readable digest on these specific issues for experts and novices alike.

Stephen M. Stahl is Adjunct Professor of Psychiatry at the University of California, San Diego and Honorary Visiting Senior Fellow in Psychiatry at the University of Cambridge, UK. He has conducted various research projects awarded by the National Institute of Mental Health, Veterans Affairs, and the pharmaceutical industry. Author of more than 500 articles and chapters, Dr Stahl is also the author of the bestsellers *Stahl's Essential Psychopharmacology* and *The Prescriber's Guide*.

Mood Disorders and Antidepressants

Stahl's Essential Psychopharmacology

Fourth Edition

Stephen M. Stahl
Adjunct Professor of Psychiatry, University of California at San Diego, California, USA
Honorary Visiting Senior Fellow in Psychiatry, University of Cambridge, Cambridge, UK

With illustrations by
Nancy Muntner

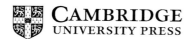
CAMBRIDGE
UNIVERSITY PRESS

CAMBRIDGE
UNIVERSITY PRESS

University Printing House, Cambridge CB2 8BS, United Kingdom

Published in the United States of America by Cambridge University Press, New York

Cambridge University Press is part of the University of Cambridge.

It furthers the University's mission by disseminating knowledge in the pursuit of education, learning and research at the highest international levels of excellence.

www.cambridge.org
Information on this title: www.cambridge.org/9781107642676

First edition published 1996
Second edition published 2000
Third edition published 2008
Fourth edition published 2013
Reprinted 2018

Printed in the United Kingdom by Print on Demand, World Wide

A catalogue record for this publication is available from the British Library

ISBN 978-1-107-64267-6

Contents

This book comprises chapters taken from *Stahl's Essential Psychopharmacology, Fourth Edition* (2013)
For further information: www.cambridge.org/9781107025981

In memory of Daniel X. Freedman, mentor, colleague, and scientific father.

To Cindy, Jennifer and Victoria

Preface

For this Mood and Antidepressants edition from the new fourth edition of *Stahl's Essential Psychopharmacology* you will notice there is a new look and feel. With a new layout, displayed over two columns, and an increased page size we have eliminated redundancies across chapters, been able to add significant new material and yet decrease the overall size of the book.

Highlights of what has been added or changed since the third edition of the textbook and the coverage of mood and antidepressants include:

– The **mood chapter** has expanded coverage of

  • stress
  • neurocircuitry
  • genetics

– The **antidepressant chapter** has:

  • new discussion and illustrations on circadian rhythms
  • discussion of the roles of neurotransmitter receptors in the mechanisms of actions of some antidepressants

    • melatonin receptors
    • 5HT1A receptors
    • 5HT2C receptors
    • 5HT3 receptors
    • 5HT7 receptors
    • NMDA glutamate receptors

  • inclusion of several new antidepressants

    • agomelatine/Valdoxan
    • vilazodone/Viibryd
    • vortioxetine (LuAA21004)
    • ketamine (rapid onset for treatment resistance)

One of the major themes emphasized in this new fourth edition is the notion of **symptom endophenotypes**, or dimensions of psychopathology that cut across numerous syndromes. This is the future of psychiatry, namely the matching of symptom endophenotypes to hypothetically malfunctioning brain circuits, regulated by genes, the environment and neurotransmitters. Hypothetically, inefficiency of information processing in these brain circuits creates symptom expression in various psychiatric disorders that can be changed with psychopharmacologic agents. Even the new DSM 5 [1] recognizes this concept and calls it Research Domain Criteria (or RDoC). Each chapter in this fourth edition discusses "symptoms and circuits" and how to exploit domains of psychopathology both to become a neurobiologically empowered psychopharmacologist, and to select and combine treatments for individual patients in psychopharmacology practice.

What has not changed in this new fourth edition is the **didactic style** of the first three editions: namely, this text attempts to present the fundamentals of psychopharmacology in **simplified and readily readable form**. We emphasize current formulations of disease mechanisms and also drug mechanisms. As in previous editions, the text is not extensively referenced to original papers, but rather to textbooks and reviews and a few selected original papers, with only a limited reading list for each chapter, but preparing the reader to consult more sophisticated textbooks as well as the professional literature.

The organization of information continues to apply the principles of **programmed learning** for the reader, namely repetition and interaction, which has been shown to enhance retention. Therefore, it is suggested that novices first approach this text by going through it from beginning to end by reviewing only the color graphics and the legends for these graphics. Virtually everything covered in the text is also covered in the graphics and icons. Once having gone through all the color graphics in these chapters, it is recommended that the reader then go back to the beginning of the book, and read the entire text, reviewing the graphics at the same time. After the text has been read, the entire book can be rapidly reviewed again merely by referring to the various color graphics in the book. This mechanism of using the materials will create a certain amount of programmed learning by incorporating the elements of repetition, as well as interaction with visual learning through graphics. Hopefully, the visual concepts learned via graphics will reinforce abstract concepts learned from the written text, especially for those of you who are primarily "visual learners," (i.e., those who retain information better from visualizing concepts than from reading about them). For those of you who are already familiar with psychopharmacology, this book should provide easy reading from beginning to end. Going back and forth between the text and the graphics should provide interaction. Following review of the complete text, it should be simple to review the entire book by going through the graphics once again.

Expansion of *Essential Psychopharmacology* Books

The fourth edition of *Essential Psychopharmacology* is the flagship, but not the entire fleet, as the *Essential Psychopharmacology* series has expanded now to an entire suite of products for the interested reader. For those of you interested in specific prescribing information, there are now three prescriber's guides:

- For psychotropic drugs, *Essential Psychopharmacology: The Prescriber's Guide*
- For neurology drugs, *Essential Neuropharmacology: The Prescriber's Guide.*
- For pain drugs: *Essential Pain Pharmacology: The Prescriber's Guide*

For those interested in how the textbook and prescriber's guides get applied in clinical practice there is a book covering 40 cases from my own clinical practice

- *Case Studies: Stahl's Essential Psychopharmacology*

For those teachers and students wanting to assess objectively their state of expertise, to pursue maintenance of certification credits for board recertification in psychiatry in the US, and for background on instructional design and how to teach there are two books:

- *Stahl's Self Assessment Examination in Psychiatry: Multiple Choice Questions for Clinicians*
- *Best Practices in Medical Teaching*

For those interested in expanded visual coverage of specialty topics in psychopharmacology, there is the *Stahl's Illustrated* series:

- *Antidepressants*
- *Antipsychotics 2nd edition: Treating Psychosis, Mania and Depression*
- *Mood Stabilizers*
- *Anxiety, Stress and PTSD*
- *Attention Deficit Hyperactivity Disorder*
- *Chronic Pain and Fibromyalgia*
- *Substance Abuse and Impulsive Disorders*

Finally, there is an ever-growing edited series of subspecialty topics:

- *Next Generation Antidepressants*
- *Essential Evidence-Based Psychopharmacology 2nd edition*
- *Essential CNS Drug Development.*

Essential Psychopharmacology Online

Now, you also have the option of accessing all these books plus additional features online by going to *Essential Psychopharmacology Online* at www. stahlonline.org. We are proud to announce the continuing update of this new Website which allows you to search online within the entire *Essential Psychopharmacology* suite of products. With publication of the fourth edition, two new features will become available on the website:

- downloadable slides of all the figures in the book
- narrated, animations of several figures in the textbook, hyperlinked to the online version of the book, playable with a click

In addition, www.stahlonline.org is now linked to:

- our new journal *CNS Spectrums*, www.journals. Cambridge.org/CNS, of which I am the new editor-in-chief, and which is now the official journal of the Neuroscience Education Institute (NEI), free online to NEI members. This journal now features readable and illustrated reviews of current topics in psychiatry, mental health, neurology and the neurosciences as well as psychopharmacology
- the NEI website, www.neiglobal.com

- for CME credits for reading the books, the journal and for completing numerous additional programs both online and live
- for access to the live course and playback encore features from the annual NEI Psychopharmacology Congress
- for access to the CME accredited NEI Master Psychopharmacology Program, an online fellowship with certification
- plans for expansion to a Cambridge University Health Partners co-accredited online Masterclass and Certificate in Psychopharmacology, based upon live programs held on campus in Cambridge and taught by University of Cambridge faculty, including myself having joined the faculty there as an Honorary Visiting Senior Fellow

Hopefully the reader can appreciate that this is an incredibly exciting time for the fields of neuroscience and mental health, creating fascinating opportunities for clinicians to utilize current therapeutics and to anticipate future medications that are likely to transform the field of psychopharmacology. Best wishes for your first step on this fascinating journey.

Stephen M. Stahl M.D, Ph.D.

1. Diagnostic and Statistical Manual of the American Psychiatric Association, in its fifth edition, new fifth edition and Research Domain Criteria (RDoC)

Mood disorders

This chapter discusses disorders characterized by abnormalities of mood: namely, depression, mania, or both. Included here are descriptions of a wide variety of mood disorders that occur over a broad clinical spectrum. Also included in this chapter is an analysis of how monoamine neurotransmitter systems are hypothetically linked to the biological basis of mood disorders. The three principal monoamine neurotransmitters are norepinephrine (NE; also called noradrenaline or NA), discussed in this chapter, dopamine (DA), discussed in Chapter 4, and serotonin (also called 5-hydroxytryptamine or 5HT), discussed in Chapter 5.

The approach taken here is to deconstruct each mood disorder into its component symptoms, followed by matching each symptom to hypothetically malfunctioning brain circuits, each regulated by one or more of the monoamine neurotransmitters. Genetic regulation and neuroimaging of these hypothetically malfunctioning brain circuits are also discussed. Coverage of symptoms and circuits of mood disorders in this chapter is intended to set the stage for understanding the pharmacological concepts underlying the mechanisms of action and use of antidepressants and mood stabilizing drugs, which will be reviewed in the following two chapters (Chapters 7 and 8).

Clinical descriptions and criteria for how to diagnose disorders of mood will only be mentioned in passing. The reader should consult standard reference sources for this material.

Description of mood disorders

Disorders of mood are often called affective disorders, since affect is the external display of mood, an emotion that is felt internally. Depression and mania are often seen as opposite ends of an affective or mood spectrum. Classically, mania and depression are "poles" apart, thus generating the terms *unipolar* depression (i.e., patients who just experience the *down* or depressed pole) and *bipolar* (i.e., patients who at different times experience either the *up* [i.e., manic] pole or the *down* [i.e., depressed] pole). Depression and mania may even occur simultaneously, which is called a *mixed* mood state. Mania may also occur in lesser degrees, known as *hypomania*, or switch so

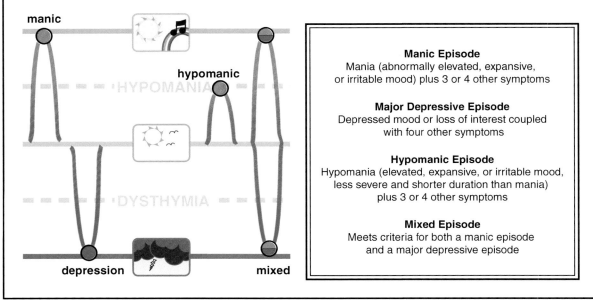

Manic Episode
Mania (abnormally elevated, expansive, or irritable mood) plus 3 or 4 other symptoms

Major Depressive Episode
Depressed mood or loss of interest coupled with four other symptoms

Hypomanic Episode
Hypomania (elevated, expansive, or irritable mood, less severe and shorter duration than mania) plus 3 or 4 other symptoms

Mixed Episode
Meets criteria for both a manic episode and a major depressive episode

Figure 6-1. Mood episodes. Bipolar disorder is generally characterized by four types of illness episodes: manic, major depressive, hypomanic, and mixed. A patient may have any combination of these episodes over the course of illness; subsyndromal manic or depressive episodes also occur during the course of illness, in which case there are not enough symptoms or the symptoms are not severe enough to meet the diagnostic criteria for one of these episodes. Thus the presentation of mood disorders can vary widely.

fast between mania and depression that it is called *rapid cycling.*

Mood disorders can be usefully visualized not only to contrast different mood disorders from one another, but also to summarize the course of illness for individual patients by showing them mapped onto a mood chart. Thus, mood ranges from hypomania to mania at the top, to euthymia (or normal mood) in the middle, to dysthymia and depression at the bottom (Figure 6-1). The most common and readily recognized mood disorder is major depressive disorder (Figure 6-2), with single or recurrent episodes. Dysthymia is a less severe but long-lasting form of depression (Figure 6-3). Patients with a major depressive episode who have poor inter-episode recovery, only to the level of dysthymia, followed by another episode of major depression are sometimes said to have "double depression," alternating between major depression and dysthymia, but not remitting (Figure 6-4).

Patients with bipolar I disorder have full-blown manic episodes or mixed episodes of mania plus depression, often followed by a depressive episode (Figure 6-5). When mania recurs at least four times a year, it is called rapid cycling (Figure 6-6A). Patients

with bipolar I disorder can also have rapid switches from mania to depression and back (Figure 6-6B). By definition, this occurs at least four times a year, but can occur much more frequently than that.

Bipolar II disorder is characterized by at least one hypomanic episode that follows a depressive episode (Figure 6-7). Cyclothymic disorder is characterized by mood swings that are not as severe as full mania and full depression, but still wax and wane above and below the boundaries of normal mood (Figure 6-8). There may be lesser degrees of variation from normal mood that are stable and persistent, including both depressive temperament (below normal mood but not a mood disorder) and hyperthymic temperament (above normal mood but also not a mood disorder) (Figure 6-9). Temperaments are personality styles of responding to environmental stimuli that can be heritable patterns present early in life and persisting throughout a lifetime; temperaments include such independent personality dimensions as novelty seeking, harm avoidance, and conscientiousness. Some patients may have mood-related temperaments, and these may render them vulnerable to mood disorders, especially bipolar spectrum disorders, later in life.

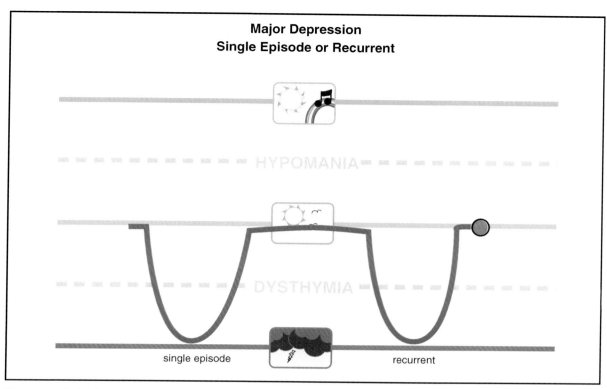

Figure 6-2. Major depression. Major depression is the most common mood disorder and is defined by the occurrence of at least a single major depressive episode, although most patients will experience recurrent episodes.

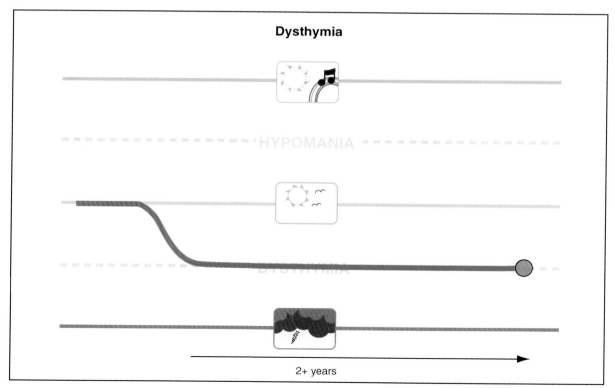

Figure 6-3. Dysthymia. Dysthymia is a less severe form of depression than major depression, but long-lasting (over 2 years in duration) and often unremitting.

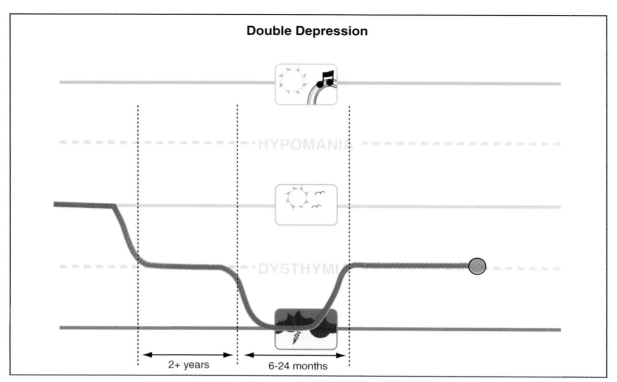

Figure 6-4. Double depression. Patients with unremitting dysthymia who also experience the superimposition of one or more major depressive episodes are described as having double depression. This is also a form of recurrent major depressive episodes with poor inter-episode recovery.

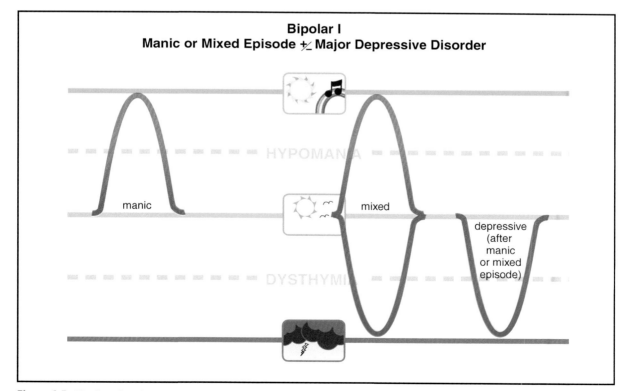

Figure 6-5. Bipolar I disorder. Bipolar I disorder is defined as the occurrence of at least one manic or mixed (full mania and full depression simultaneously) episode. Patients with bipolar I disorder typically experience major depressive episodes as well, although this is not necessary for the bipolar I diagnosis.

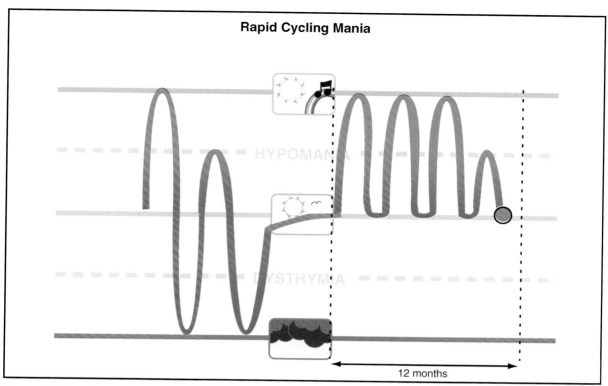

Figure 6-6A. Rapid cycling mania. The course of bipolar disorder can be rapid cycling, which means that at least four episodes occur within a 1-year period. This can manifest itself as four distinct manic episodes, as shown here. Many patients with this form of mood disorder experience switches much more frequently than four times a year.

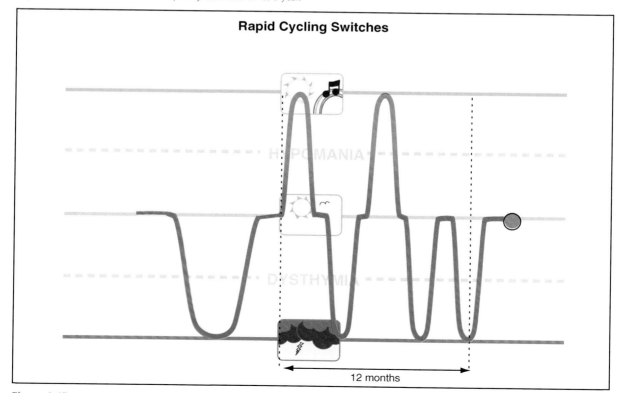

Figure 6-6B. Rapid cycling switches. A rapid cycling course (at least four distinct mood episodes within 1 year) can also manifest as rapid switches between manic and depressive episodes.

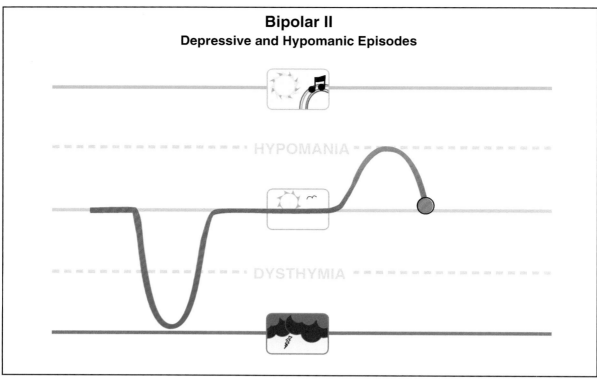

Figure 6-7. Bipolar II disorder. Bipolar II disorder is defined as an illness course consisting of one or more major depressive episodes and at least one hypomanic episode.

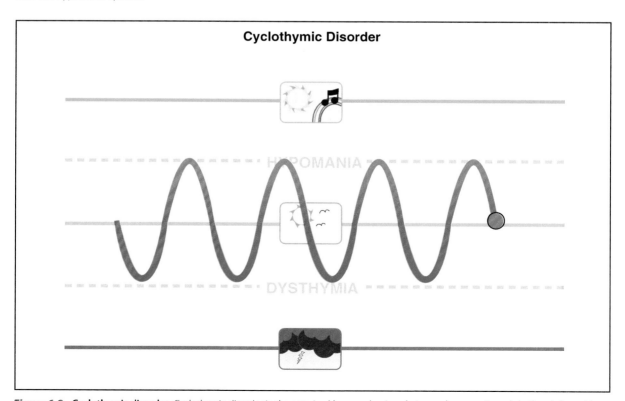

Figure 6-8. Cyclothymic disorder. Cyclothymic disorder is characterized by mood swings between hypomania and dysthymia but without any full manic or major depressive episodes.

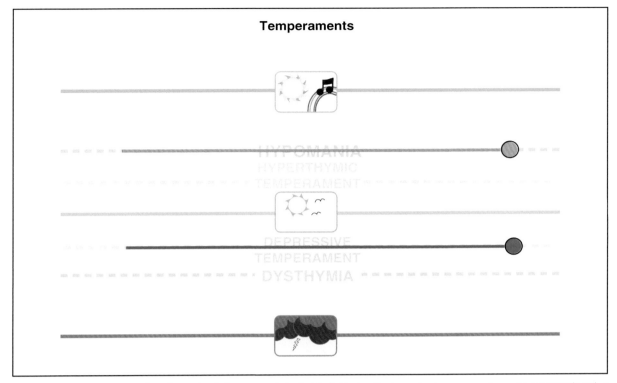

Figure 6-9. Temperaments. Not all mood variations are pathological. Individuals with depressive temperament may be consistently sad or apathetic but do not meet the criteria for dysthymia and do not necessarily experience any functional impairment. However, individuals with depressive temperament may be at greater risk for the development of a mood disorder later in life. Hyperthymic temperament, in which mood is above normal but not pathological, includes stable characteristics such as extroversion, optimism, exuberance, impulsiveness, overconfidence, grandiosity, and lack of inhibition. Individuals with hyperthymic temperament may be at greater risk for the development of a mood disorder later in life.

The bipolar spectrum

From a strict diagnostic point of view, our discussion of mood disorders could now be mostly complete. However, there is the growing recognition that many patients seen in clinical practice have a mood disorder not well described by the above categories. Formally, they would be called "not otherwise specified" or "NOS," but this creates a huge single category for many patients that belies the richness and complexity of their symptoms. Increasingly, such patients are seen as belonging in general to the "bipolar spectrum" (Figure 6-10), and in particular to one of several additional descriptive categories that have been proposed by experts such as Hagop Akiskal (Figures 6-10 through 6-20).

Bipolar ¼ (0.25)

One mood disorder often considered to be "not quite bipolar" and sometimes called bipolar ¼ (or 0.25) designates an unstable form of unipolar depression that

responds sometimes rapidly but in an unsustained manner to antidepressants, the latter sometimes called antidepressant "poop-out" (Figure 6-11). These patients have unstable mood but not a formal bipolar disorder, yet can benefit from mood-stabilizing treatments added to robust antidepressant treatments.

Bipolar ½ (0.5) and schizoaffective disorder

Another type of mood disorder is called different things by different experts, from bipolar ½ (or 0.5) to "schizobipolar disorder" to "schizoaffective disorder" (Figure 6-12). For over a century, experts have debated whether psychotic disorders are dichotomous from mood disorders (Figure 6-13A) or are part of a continuous disease spectrum from psychosis to mood (Figure 6-13B).

The dichotomous disease model is in the tradition of Kraepelin and proposes that schizophrenia is a chronic unremitting illness with poor outcome and decline in

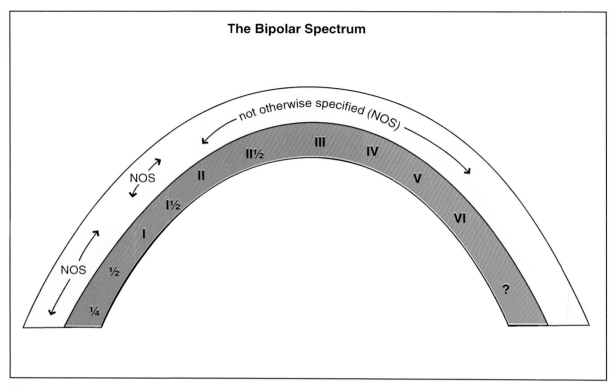

Figure 6-10. Bipolar spectrum. There is a huge variation in the presentation of patients with bipolar disorder. Historically, bipolar disorder has been categorized as I, II, or not otherwise specified (NOS). It may be more useful, instead, to think of these patients as belonging to a bipolar spectrum and to identify subcategories of presentations, as has been done by Akiskal and other experts and as illustrated in the next several figures.

function whereas bipolar disorder is a cyclical illness with a better outcome and good restoration of function between episodes. However, there is great debate as to how to define the borders between these two illnesses. One notion is that cases with overlapping symptoms and intermediate disease courses can be seen as a third illness, schizoaffective disorder. Today, many define this border with the idea that "even a trace of schizophrenia is schizophrenia." From this "schizophrenia-centered perspective," many overlapping cases of psychotic mania and psychotic depression might be considered either to be forms of schizophrenia, or to be schizoaffective disorder as a form of schizophrenia with affective symptoms. A competing point of view within the dichotomous model is that "even a trace of mood disturbance is a mood disorder." From this "mood-centered perspective," many overlapping cases of psychotic mania and psychotic depression might be considered either to be forms of a mood/bipolar disorder or to be schizoaffective disorder as a form of mood/bipolar disorder with psychotic symptoms. Where

patients have a mixture of mood symptoms and psychosis, it can obviously be very difficult to tell whether they have a psychotic disorder such as schizophrenia, a mood disorder such as bipolar disorder, or a third condition, schizoaffective disorder. Some even want to eliminate the diagnosis of schizoaffective disorder entirely.

Proponents of the dichotomous model point out that treatments for schizophrenia differ from those for bipolar disorder, since lithium is rarely helpful in schizophrenia, and anticonvulsant mood stabilizers have limited efficacy for psychotic symptoms in schizophrenia, and perhaps only as augmenting agents. Treatments for schizoaffective disorder can include both treatments for schizophrenia and treatments for bipolar disorder. The current debate within the dichotomous model is: If you have bipolar disorder, do you have a good outcome? – but if you have schizophrenia, do you have a poor outcome? – and what genetic and biological markers rather than clinical symptoms can distinguish one dichotomous entity from the other?

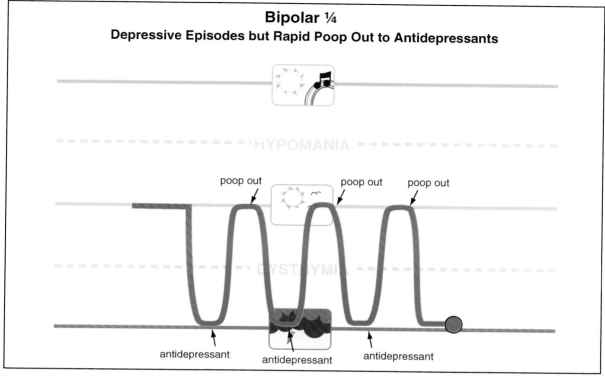

Figure 6-11. Bipolar ¼. Some patients may present only with depressive symptoms yet exhibit rapid but unsustained response to antidepressant treatment (sometimes called rapid "poop out"). Although such patients may have no spontaneous mood symptoms above normal, they potentially could benefit from mood-stabilizing treatment. This presentation may be termed bipolar ¼ (or bipolar 0.25).

The continuum disease model proposes that psychotic and mood disorders are both manifestations of one complex set of disorders that is expressed across a spectrum, at one end schizophrenia (plus schizophreniform disorder, brief psychotic disorder, delusional disorder, shared psychotic disorder, subsyndromal/ultra-high-risk psychosis prodrome, schizotypal, paranoid, schizoid, and even avoidant personality disorders), and at the other end bipolar/mood disorders (mania, depression, mixed states, melancholic depression, atypical depression, catatonic depression, postpartum depression, psychotic depression, seasonal affective disorder), with schizoaffective disorder in the middle, combining features of positive symptoms of psychosis with manic, hypomanic, or depressive episodes (Figure 6-13B).

Modern genomics suggests that the spectrum is not a single disease, but a complex of hundreds if not thousands of different diseases, with overlapping genetic, epigenetic, and biomarkers as well as overlapping clinical symptoms and functional outcomes. Proponents of the continuum model point out that treatments for schizophrenia overlap greatly now with those for bipolar disorder, since second-generation atypical antipsychotics are effective in the positive symptoms of schizophrenia and in psychotic mania and psychotic depression, and are also effective in nonpsychotic mania and in bipolar depression and unipolar depression. These same second-generation atypical antipsychotics are effective for the spectrum of symptoms in schizoaffective disorder. From the continuum disease perspective, failure to give mood-stabilizing medications may lead to suboptimal symptom relief in patients with psychosis, even those whose prominent or eye-catching psychotic symptoms mask or distract clinicians from seeing underlying and perhaps more subtle mood symptoms. In the continuum disease model, schizophrenia can be seen as the extreme end of a spectrum of severity of mood disorders and not a disease unrelated to a mood disorder. Schizophrenia can therefore share with schizoaffective disorder severe psychotic symptoms that obscure mood symptoms, a chronic course that eliminates cycling, resistance to antipsychotic treatments, and prominent

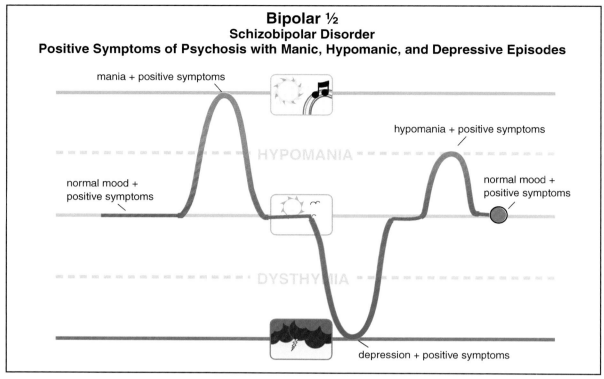

Bipolar ½
Schizobipolar Disorder
Positive Symptoms of Psychosis with Manic, Hypomanic, and Depressive Episodes

mania + positive symptoms

hypomania + positive symptoms

HYPOMANIA

normal mood +
positive symptoms

normal mood +
positive symptoms

DYSTHYMIA

depression + positive symptoms

Figure 6-12. Bipolar ½. Bipolar ½ (0.5) has been described as schizobipolar disorder, which combines positive symptoms of psychosis with manic, hypomanic, and depressive episodes.

Schizophrenia and Bipolar Disorder

Dichotomous Disease Model

Schizophrenia	Schizoaffective Disorder	Bipolar Disorder
• psychosis	• psychosis	• mania
• chronic, unremitting	and	• mood disorder
• poor outcome	• mania	• cyclical
• "even a trace of schizophrenia is schizophrenia"	• mood disorder	• good outcome
		• "even a trace of a mood disturbance is a mood disorder"

Figure 6-13A. Schizophrenia and bipolar disorder: dichotomous disease model. Schizophrenia and bipolar disorder have been conceptualized both as dichotomous disorders and as belonging to a continuum. In the dichotomous disease model, schizophrenia consists of chronic, unremitting psychosis, with poor outcomes expected. Bipolar disorder consists of cyclical manic and other mood episodes and has better expected outcomes than schizophrenia. A third distinct disorder is schizoaffective disorder, characterized by psychosis and mania as well as other mood symptoms.

Schizophrenia and Bipolar Disorder

Continuum Disease Model

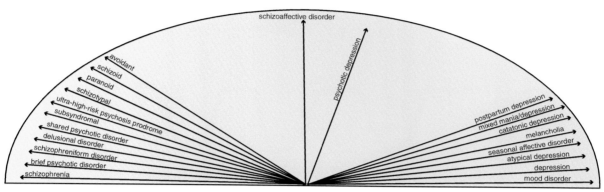

Figure 6-13B. Schizophrenia and bipolar disorder: continuum disease model. Schizophrenia and bipolar disorder have been conceptualized both as dichotomous disorders and as belonging to a continuum. In the continuum disease model, schizophrenia and mood disorders fall along a continuum in which psychosis, delusions, and paranoid avoidant behavior are on one extreme and depression and other mood symptoms are on the other extreme. Falling in the middle are psychotic depression and schizoaffective disorder.

negative symptoms, yet be just a severe form of the same illness. In the continuum disease model, schizoaffective disorder would be a milder form of the illness with less severe psychotic features and more severe mood features.

The debate rages on . . .

Bipolar I½ (1.5)

Although patients with protracted or recurrent hypomania without depression are not formally diagnosed as bipolar II disorder, they are definitely part of the bipolar spectrum, and may benefit from mood stabilizers that have been studied mostly in bipolar I disorder (Figure 6-14). Eventually, such patients will often develop a major depressive episode and their diagnosis will then change to bipolar II disorder, but in the meantime they can be treated for hypomania while being vigilant to the future onset of a major depressive episode.

Bipolar II½ (2.5)

Bipolar II½ is the designation for cyclothymic patients who develop major depressive episodes (Figure 6-15). Many patients with cyclothymia are just considered "moody" and do not consult professionals until experiencing full depressive episodes. It is important to recognize patients in this part of the bipolar spectrum, because treatment of their major

depressive episodes with antidepressant monotherapy may actually cause increased mood cycling or even induction of a full manic episode, just as can happen in patients with bipolar I or II depressive episodes.

Bipolar III (3.0)

Patients who develop a manic or hypomanic episode on an antidepressant are sometimes called bipolar III (Figure 6-16). According to formal diagnostic criteria, however, when an antidepressant causes mania or hypomania, the diagnosis is not bipolar disorder, but rather, "substance-induced mood disorder." Many experts disagree with this designation and feel that patients who have a hypomanic or manic response to an antidepressant do so because they have a bipolar spectrum disorder, and can be more appropriately diagnosed as bipolar III disorder (Figure 6-16) until they experience a spontaneous manic or hypomanic episode while taking no drugs, at which point their diagnosis would be bipolar I or II, respectively. The bipolar III designation is helpful in the meantime, reminding clinicians that such patients are not good candidates for antidepressant monotherapy.

Bipolar III½ (3.5)

A variant of this bipolar III disorder has been called bipolar III½, to designate a type of bipolar disorder associated with substance abuse (Figure 6-17).

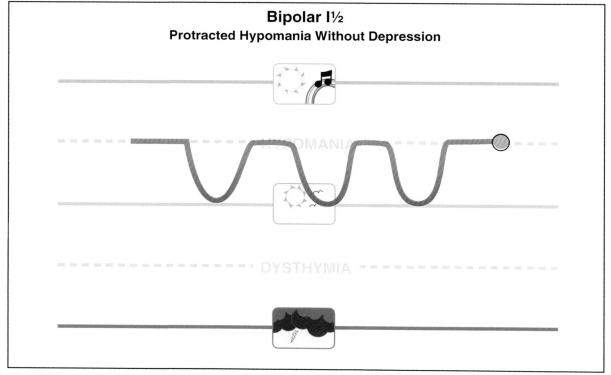

Figure 6-14. Bipolar I½. A formal diagnosis of bipolar II disorder requires the occurrence of not only hypomanic episodes but also depressive episodes. However, some patients may experience recurrent hypomania without having experienced a depressive episode – a presentation that may be termed bipolar I½. These patients may be at risk of eventually developing a depressive episode and are candidates for mood-stabilizing treatment, although no treatment is formally approved for this condition.

Although some of these patients can utilize substances of abuse to treat depressive episodes, others have previously experienced natural or drug-induced mania and take substances of abuse to induce mania. This combination of a bipolar disorder with substance abuse is a formula for chaos, and can often be the story of a patient prior to seeking treatment from a mental health professional.

Bipolar IV (4.0)

Bipolar IV disorder is the association of depressive episodes with a pre-existing hyperthymic temperament (Figure 6-18). Patients with hyperthymia are often sunny, optimistic, high-output, successful individuals with stable temperament for years and then suddenly collapse into a severe depression. In such cases, it may be useful to be vigilant to the need for more than antidepressant monotherapy if the patient is unresponsive to such treatment, or if the patient develops rapid cycling or hypomanic or mixed states in response to antidepressants. Despite not having a

formal bipolar disorder, such patients may respond best to mood stabilizers.

Bipolar V (5.0)

Bipolar V disorder is depression with mixed hypomania (Figure 6-19). Formal diagnostic criteria for mixed states require full expression of both depression and mania simultaneously, but in the real world, many depressed patients can have additional symptoms that only qualify as hypomania or subsyndromal hypomania, or even just a few manic symptoms or only mild manic symptoms. Depression simultaneous with full hypomania is represented in Figure 6-1 and Figure 6-5 and requires mood stabilizer treatment, not antidepressant monotherapy. Under debate is whether there should be a separate diagnostic category for depression with subthreshold hypomania; some experts believe that up to half of patients with major depression also have a lifetime history of subsyndromal hypomania, and that these patients are much more likely to progress to a formal bipolar

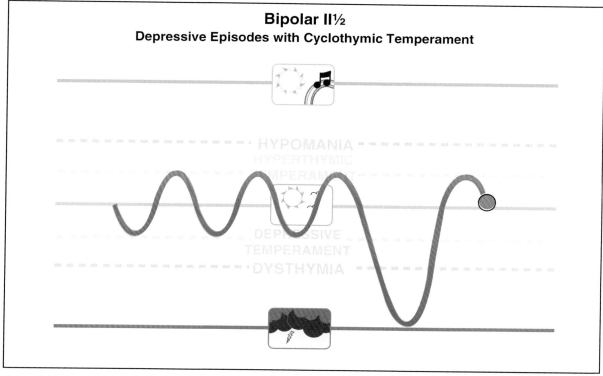

Figure 6-15. Bipolar II½. Patients may present with a major depressive episode in the context of cyclothymic temperament, which is characterized by oscillations between hyperthymic or hypomanic states (above normal) and depressive or dysthymic states (below normal) upon which a major depressive episode intrudes (bipolar II½). Individuals with cyclothymic temperament who are treated for the major depressive episodes may be at increased risk for antidepressant-induced mood cycling.

diagnosis. Patients with depression and subthreshold hypomania generally have a worse outcome, more mood episodes, more work impairment, are more likely to have a family member with mania or other bipolar disorder, and to have an early onset of depression. For depression with subsyndromal hypomania it may be more important to emphasize overactivity rather than just mood elevation, and a duration of only 2 days as opposed to the 4 days required in most diagnostic systems for hypomania. Whether these patients can be treated with antidepressant monotherapy without precipitating mania, or instead require agents with potentially greater side effects such as mood stabilizers, lithium, and/or atypical antipsychotics, is still under investigation.

Related conditions to depression mixed with subsyndromal hypomania include other mood states where full diagnostic criteria are not reached, ranging from full mixed states (both full mania diagnostic criteria [M] and full depression diagnostic criteria [D]) to depression with hypomania or only a few hypomanic symptoms (mD) as already discussed. In addition, other combinations of mania and depression range from full mania with only a few depressive symptoms (Md, sometimes also called "dysphoric" mania), to subsyndromal but unstable states characterized by some symptoms of both mania and depression, but not diagnostic of either (md) (Table 6-1). All of these states differ from unipolar depression and belong in the bipolar spectrum; they may require treatment with the same agents that are used to treat bipolar I or II disorder, with appropriate caution for antidepressant monotherapy. Just because a patient is depressed, it does not mean he or she should start with an antidepressant for treatment. Patients with mixed states of depression and mania may be particularly vulnerable to the induction of activation, agitation, rapid cycling, dysphoria, hypomania, mania, or suicidality when treated with antidepressants, particularly without the concomitant use of a mood stabilizer or an atypical antipsychotic.

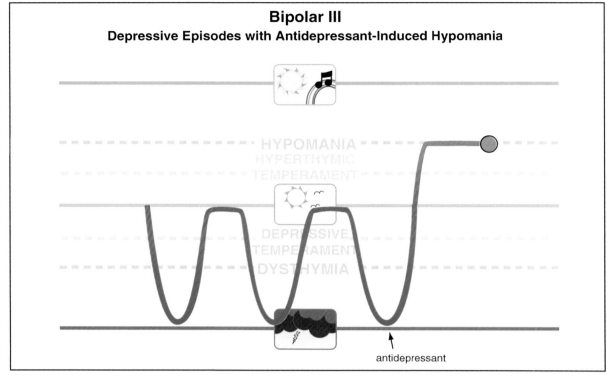

Bipolar III
Depressive Episodes with Antidepressant-Induced Hypomania

Figure 6-16. Bipolar III. Although the *Diagnostic and Statistical Manual of Mental Disorders*, fourth edition (DSM-IV), defines antidepressant-induced (hypo)mania as a substance-induced mood disorder, some experts believe that individuals who experience substance-induced (hypo)mania are actually predisposed to these mood states and thus belong to the bipolar spectrum (bipolar III).

Bipolar VI (6.0)

Finally, bipolar VI disorder (Figure 6-20) represents bipolarity in the setting of dementia, where it can be incorrectly attributed to the behavioral symptoms of dementia rather than recognized and treated as a comorbid mood state with mood stabilizers and even with atypical antipsychotics.

Many more subtypes of mood disorders can be described within the bipolar spectrum. The important thing to take away from this discussion is that not all patients with depression have major depressive disorder requiring treatment with antidepressant monotherapy, and that there are many states of mood disorder within the bipolar spectrum beyond just bipolar I and II disorders.

Can unipolar depression be distinguished from bipolar depression?

One of the important developments in the field of mood disorders in recent years in fact is the recognition that many patients once considered to have major depressive disorder actually have a form of bipolar disorder, especially bipolar II disorder or one of the conditions within the bipolar spectrum (Figure 6-21). Since symptomatic patients with bipolar disorder spend much more of their time in the depressed state rather than in the manic, hypomanic, or mixed state, this means that many depressed patients in the past were incorrectly diagnosed with unipolar major depression, and treated with antidepressant monotherapy instead of being diagnosed as a bipolar spectrum disorder and treated first with lithium, anticonvulsant mood stabilizers, and/or atypical antipsychotics prior to adding an antidepressant, if an antidepressant is even used at all.

Up to half of patients once considered to have a unipolar depression are now considered to have a bipolar spectrum disorder (Figure 6-21), and although they would not necessarily be good candidates for antidepressant monotherapy, this is often the treatment that they receive when the bipolar nature of their condition is not recognized. Antidepressant treatment of unrecognized bipolar patients

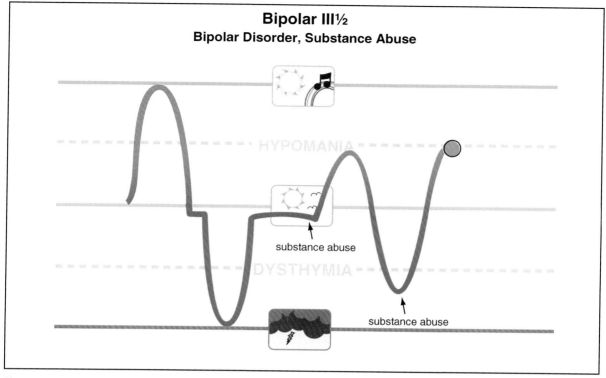

Figure 6-17. Bipolar III½. Bipolar III½ (3.5) is bipolar disorder with substance abuse, in which the substance abuse is associated with efforts to achieve hypomania. Such patients should be evaluated closely to determine if (hypo)mania has ever occurred in the absence of substance abuse.

may not only increase mood cycling, mixed states, and conversion to hypomania and mania, as mentioned above, but may also contribute to the increase in suicidality in younger patients treated with antidepressants, i.e., children and adults younger than 25.

Thus it becomes important to recognize whether a depressed patient has a bipolar spectrum disorder or a unipolar major depressive disorder. How can this be done? In reality, patients with either unipolar or bipolar depression often have identical current symptoms, so obtaining the profile of current symptomatology is obviously not sufficient for distinguishing unipolar from bipolar depression. The answer may be in part to ask the two questions shown in Table 6-2, namely, "Who's your daddy?" and "Where's your mama?"

"Who's your daddy?" can mean "what is your family history?" since a first-degree relative with a bipolar spectrum disorder can give a strong hint that the patient also has a bipolar spectrum disorder rather than unipolar depression. "Where's your mama?" can mean "I need to get additional history from someone

else close to you," since patients tend to under-report their manic symptoms, and the insight and observations of an outside informant such as a mother or spouse can describe a history quite different from the one the patient is reporting, and thus help establish a bipolar spectrum diagnosis that patients themselves do not perceive, or deny. Some hints, but not sufficient for diagnostic certainty, can even come from current symptoms to suggest a bipolar spectrum depression, such as more time sleeping, overeating, comorbid anxiety, motor retardation, mood lability, psychotic symptoms or suicidal thoughts (Figure 6-22). Hints that the depression may be in the bipolar spectrum can also come from the course of the untreated illness prior to the current symptoms, such as early age of onset, high frequency of depressive symptoms, high proportion of time spent ill, and acute abatement or onset of symptoms. Prior response to antidepressants that suggests bipolar depression can be multiple antidepressant failures, rapid recovery, and activating side effects such as

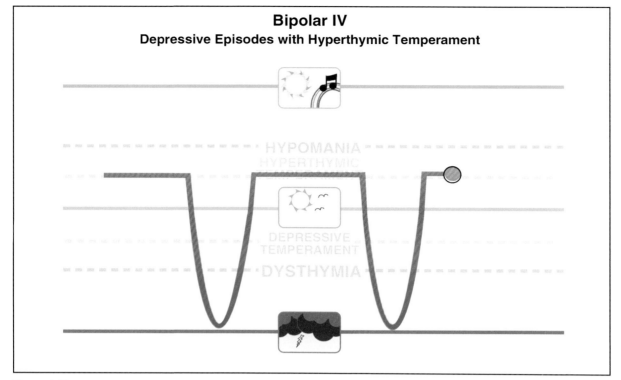

Figure 6-18. Bipolar IV. Bipolar IV is seen in individuals with longstanding and stable hyperthymic temperament into which a major depressive episode intrudes. Individuals with hyperthymic temperament who are treated for depressive episodes may be at increased risk for antidepressant-induced mood cycling, and may instead respond better to mood stabilizers.

insomnia, agitation, and anxiety. Although none of these features can discriminate bipolar depression from unipolar depression with certainty, the point is to be vigilant to the possibility that what looks like a unipolar depression might actually be a bipolar spectrum depression when investigated more carefully, and when response to treatment is monitored.

Are mood disorders progressive?

One of the major unanswered questions about the natural history of depressive illnesses is whether they are progressive (Figures 6-23 and 6-24). Some observers believe that there is an increasing number of patients in mental health practices who have bipolar spectrum illnesses rather than unipolar illnesses, especially compared to a few decades ago. Is this merely the product of changing diagnostic criteria, or does unipolar depression progress to bipolar depression (Figure 6-23)? A corollary of this question is whether chronic and widespread undertreatment of unipolar depression,

allowing residual symptoms to persist and relapses and recurrences to occur, results first in more rapidly recurring episodes of major depression, then in poor inter-episode recovery, then progression to a bipolar spectrum condition, and finally to treatment resistance (Figure 6-23). Many treatment-resistant mood disorders in psychiatric practices have elements of bipolar spectrum disorder that can be identified, and many of these patients require treatment with more than antidepressants, or with mood stabilizers and atypical antipsychotics instead of antidepressants. For patients already diagnosed with bipolar disorder, there is similar concern that the disorder may be progressive, especially without adequate treatment. Thus, discrete manic and depressive episodes may progress to mixed and dysphoric episodes, and finally to rapid cycling, instability, and treatment resistance (Figure 6-24). The hope is that recognition and treatment of both unipolar and bipolar depressions, causing all symptoms to remit for long periods of time, might prevent progression to more difficult states. This is not proven, but is a major

Table 6-1 Mixed states of mania and depression

Description	Designation	Comment
DSM-IV mixed	MD	Full diagnostic criteria for both mania and depression
Depression with hypomania	mD	Bipolar V
Depression with some manic symptoms	mD	Bipolar NOS
Mania with some depressive symptoms	Md	Dysphoric mania
Subsyndromal mania and subsyndromal depression	md	Prodrome or presymptomatic state of incomplete remission

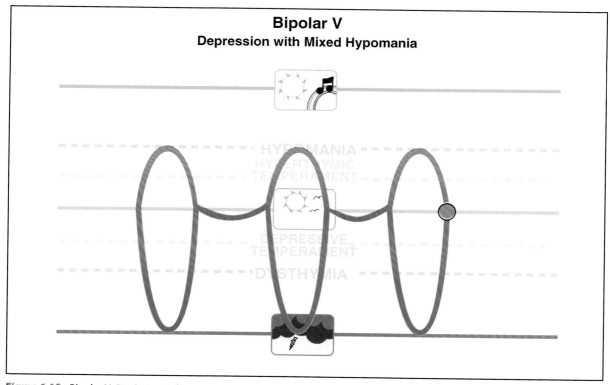

Bipolar V
Depression with Mixed Hypomania

Figure 6-19. Bipolar V. Bipolar V is defined as major depressive episodes with hypomanic symptoms occurring during the major depressive episode but without the presence of discrete hypomanic episodes. Because the symptoms do not meet the full criteria for mania, these patients would not be considered to have a full mixed episode, but they nonetheless exhibit a mixed presentation and may require mood stabilizer treatment as opposed to antidepressant monotherapy.

hypothesis in the field at the present time. In the meantime, practitioners must decide whether to commit "sins of omission," and be conservative with the diagnosis of bipolar spectrum disorder, and err on the side of undertreatment of mood disorders, or "sins of commission," and overdiagnose and overtreat symptoms in the hope that this will prevent disease progression.

Neurotransmitters and circuits in mood disorders

Three principal neurotransmitters have long been implicated in both the pathophysiology and treatment of mood disorders. They are norepinephrine, dopamine, and serotonin, and comprise what is sometimes called

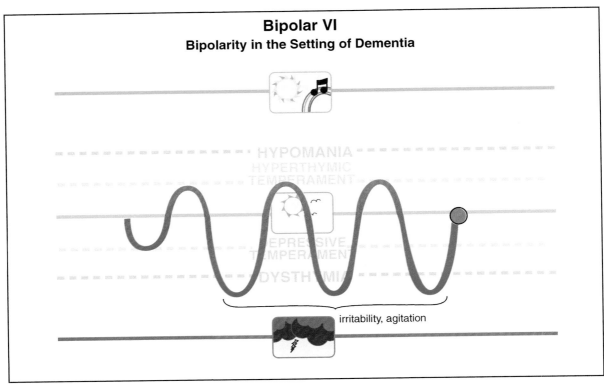

Figure 6-20. Bipolar VI. Another subcategory within the bipolar spectrum may be "bipolarity in the setting of dementia," termed bipolar VI. Mood instability here begins late in life, followed by impaired attention, irritability, reduced drive, and disrupted sleep. The presentation may initially appear to be attributable to dementia or be considered unipolar depression, but it is likely to be exacerbated by antidepressants and may respond to mood stabilizers.

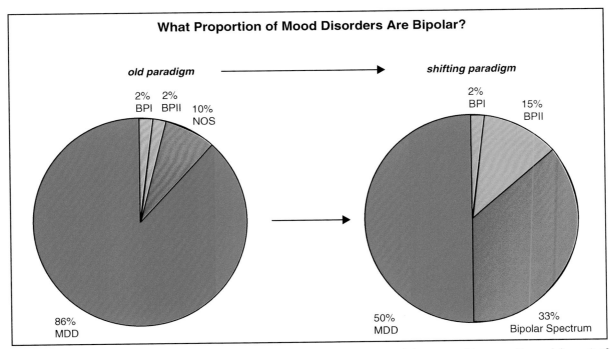

Figure 6-21. Prevalence of mood disorders. In recent years there has been a paradigm shift in terms of the recognition and diagnosis of patients with mood disorders. That is, many patients once considered to have major depressive disorder (old paradigm, left) are now recognized as having bipolar II disorder or another form of bipolar illness within the bipolar spectrum (shifting paradigm, right).

Table 6-2 Is it unipolar or bipolar depression? Questions to ask

Who's your daddy?

What is your family history of:

- mood disorder?
- psychiatric hospitalizations?
- suicide?
- anyone who took lithium, mood stabilizers, antipsychotics, antidepressants?
- anyone who received ECT?

These can be indications of a unipolar or bipolar spectrum disorder in relatives.

Where's your mama?

I need to get additional history about you from someone close to you, such as your mother or your spouse.

Patients may especially lack insight about their manic symptoms and under-report them.

the monoamine neurotransmitter system. These three monoamines often work in concert. Many of the symptoms of mood disorders are hypothesized to involve dysfunction of various combinations of these three systems. Essentially all known treatments for mood disorders act upon one or more of these three systems.

We have extensively discussed the dopamine system in Chapter 4 and illustrated it in Figures 4-5 through 4-11. We have extensively discussed the serotonin system in Chapter 5 and illustrated it in Figures 5-13, 5-14, 5-25, and 5-27. Here we introduce the reader to the norepinephrine system, and also show some interactions among these three monoaminergic neurotransmitter systems.

Noradrenergic neurons

The noradrenergic neuron utilizes norepinephrine (noradrenaline) as its neurotransmitter. Norepinephrine (NE) is synthesized, or produced, from the precursor

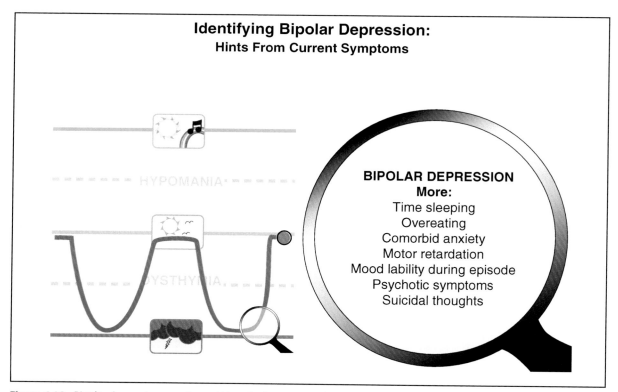

Figure 6-22. Bipolar depression symptoms. Although all symptoms of a major depressive episode can occur in either unipolar or bipolar depression, some symptoms may present more often in bipolar versus unipolar depression, providing hints if not diagnostic certainty that the patient has a bipolar spectrum disorder. These symptoms include increased time sleeping, overeating, comorbid anxiety, psychomotor retardation, mood lability during episodes, psychotic symptoms, and suicidal thoughts.

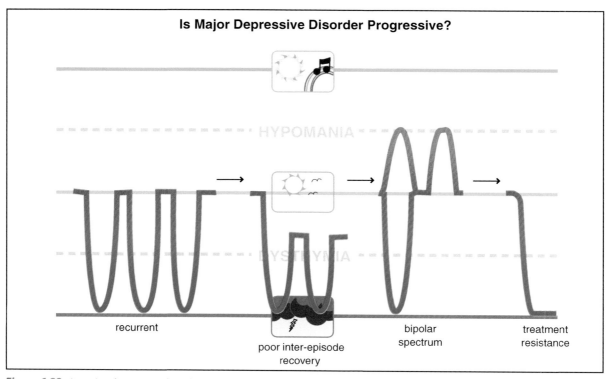

Figure 6-23. Is major depressive disorder progressive? A currently unanswered question is whether mood disorders are progressive. Does undertreatment of unipolar depression, in which residual symptoms persist and relapses occur, lead to progressive worsening of illness, such as more frequent recurrences and poor inter-episode recovery? And can this ultimately progress to a bipolar spectrum condition and finally treatment resistance?

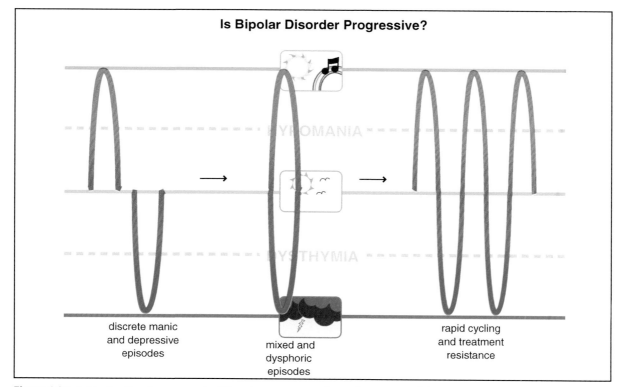

Figure 6-24. Is bipolar disorder progressive? There is some concern that undertreatment of discrete manic and depressive episodes may progress to mixed and dysphoric episodes and finally to rapid cycling and treatment resistance.

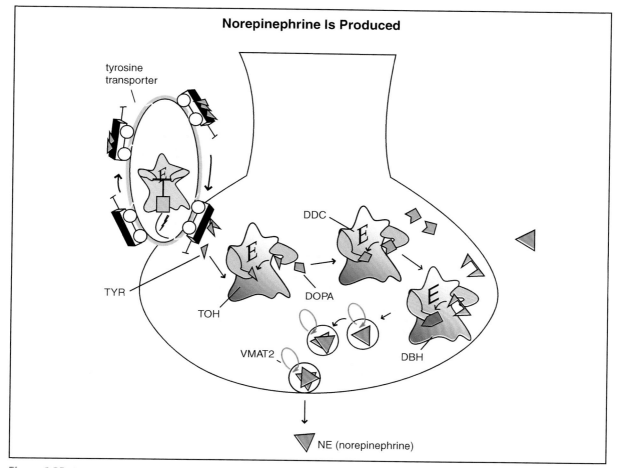

Figure 6-25. Norepinephrine is produced. Tyrosine (TYR) a precursor to norepinephrine (NE), is taken up into NE nerve terminals via a tyrosine transporter and converted into DOPA by the enzyme tyrosine hydroxylase (TOH). DOPA is then converted into dopamine (DA) by the enzyme DOPA decarboxylase (DDC). Finally, DA is converted into NE by dopamine β-hydroxylase (DBH). After synthesis, NE is packaged into synaptic vesicles via the vesicular monoamine transporter (VMAT2) and stored there until its release into the synapse during neurotransmission.

amino acid tyrosine, which is transported into the nervous system from the blood by means of an active transport pump (Figure 6-25). Once inside the neuron, the tyrosine is acted upon by three enzymes in sequence. First, tyrosine hydroxylase (TOH), the rate-limiting and most important enzyme in the regulation of NE synthesis. Tyrosine hydroxylase converts the amino acid tyrosine into DOPA. The second enzyme then acts, namely, DOPA decarboxylase (DDC), which converts DOPA into dopamine (DA). DA itself is a neurotransmitter in dopamine neurons, as discussed in Chapter 4 and illustrated in Figure 4-5. However, for NE neurons, DA is just a precursor of NE. In fact the third and final NE synthetic enzyme, dopamine β-hydroxylase (DBH), converts DA into NE. NE is then stored in synaptic

packages called vesicles until released by a nerve impulse (Figure 6-25).

NE action is terminated by two principal destructive or catabolic enzymes that turn NE into inactive metabolites. The first is monoamine oxidase (MAO) A or B, which is located in mitochondria in the presynaptic neuron and elsewhere (Figure 6-26). The second is catechol-O-methyl-transferase (COMT), which is thought to be located largely outside of the presynaptic nerve terminal (Figure 6-26).

The action of NE can be terminated not only by enzymes that destroy NE, but also by a transport pump for NE that removes NE from acting in the synapse without destroying it (Figure 6-27). In fact, such inactivated NE can be restored for reuse in a later

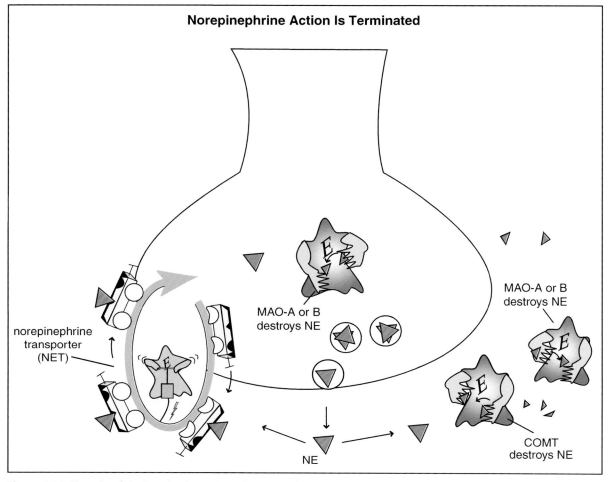

Figure 6-26. Norepinephrine's action is terminated. Norepinephrine's action can be terminated through multiple mechanisms. Dopamine can be transported out of the synaptic cleft and back into the presynaptic neuron via the norepinephrine transporter (NET), where it may be repackaged for future use. Alternatively, norepinephrine may be broken down extracellularly via the enzyme catechol-*O*-methyl-transferase (COMT). Other enzymes that break down norepinephrine are monoamine oxidase A (MAO-A) and monoamine oxidase B (MAO-B), which are present in mitochondria both within the presynaptic neuron and in other cells, including neurons and glia.

neurotransmitting nerve impulse. The transport pump that terminates synaptic action of NE is sometimes called the "NE transporter" or NET and sometimes the "NE reuptake pump." This NE reuptake pump is located on the presynaptic noradrenergic nerve terminal as part of the presynaptic machinery of the neuron, where it acts as a vacuum cleaner whisking NE out of the synapse, off the synaptic receptors, and stopping its synaptic actions. Once inside the presynaptic nerve terminal, NE can either be stored again for subsequent reuse when another nerve impulse arrives, or destroyed by NE-destroying enzymes (Figure 6-26).

The noradrenergic neuron is regulated by a multiplicity of receptors for NE (Figure 6-27). The norepinephrine transporter or NET is one type of receptor, as is the vesicular monoamine transporter (VMAT2) that transports NE in the cytoplasm of the presynaptic neuron into storage vesicles (Figure 6-27). NE receptors are classified as α_1 or α_{2A}, α_{2B}, or α_{2C}, or as β_1, β_2, or β_3. All can be postsynaptic, but only α_2 receptors can act as presynaptic autoreceptors (Figures 6-27 through 6-29). Postsynaptic receptors convert their occupancy by norepinephrine at α_1, α_{2A}, α_{2B}, α_{2C}, β_1, β_2, or β_3 receptors into physiological functions, and ultimately into

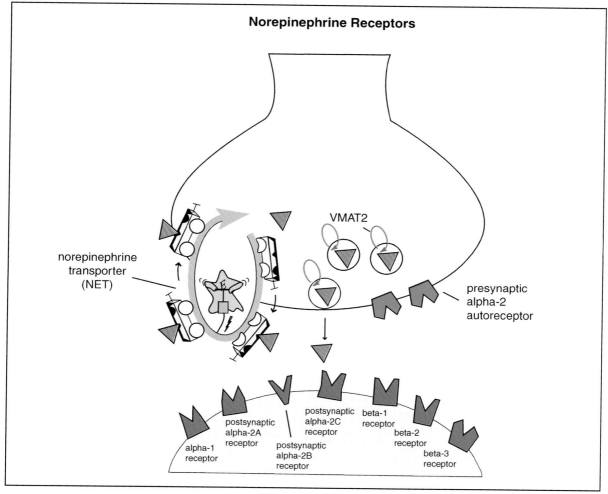

Figure 6-27. Norepinephrine receptors. Shown here are receptors for norepinephrine that regulate its neurotransmission. The norepinephrine transporter (NET) exists presynaptically and is responsible for clearing excess norepinephrine out of the synapse. The vesicular monoamine transporter (VMAT2) takes norepinephrine up into synaptic vesicles and stores it for future neurotransmission. There is also a presynaptic α_2 autoreceptor, which regulates release of norepinephrine from the presynaptic neuron. In addition, there are several postsynaptic receptors. These include α_1, α_{2A}, α_{2B}, α_{2C}, β_1, β_2, and β_3 receptors.

changes in signal transduction and gene expression in the postsynaptic neuron (Figure 6-27).

Presynaptic α_2 receptors regulate norepinephrine release, so they are called *autoreceptors* (Figures 6-27 and 6-28). Presynaptic α_2 autoreceptors are located both on the axon terminal (i.e., terminal α_2 receptors: Figures 6-27 and 6-28) and at cell body (soma) and nearby dendrities; thus, these latter α_2 presynapic receptors are called *somatodendritic* α_2 receptors (Figure 6-29). Presynaptic α_2 receptors are important because both the terminal and the somatodendritic α_2 receptors are autoreceptors. That is, when presynaptic α_2 receptors recognize NE, they turn off further release of NE (Figures 6-27 and 6-28). Thus, presynaptic α_2 autoreceptors act as a brake for the NE neuron, and also cause what is known as a negative-feedback regulatory signal. Stimulating this receptor (i.e., stepping on the brake) stops the neuron from firing. This probably occurs physiologically to prevent over-firing of the NE neuron, since it can shut itself off once the firing rate gets too high and the autoreceptor becomes stimulated. It is worthy to note that drugs can not only mimic the natural functioning of the NE neuron by stimulating the presynaptic α_2 neuron, but drugs that antagonize this

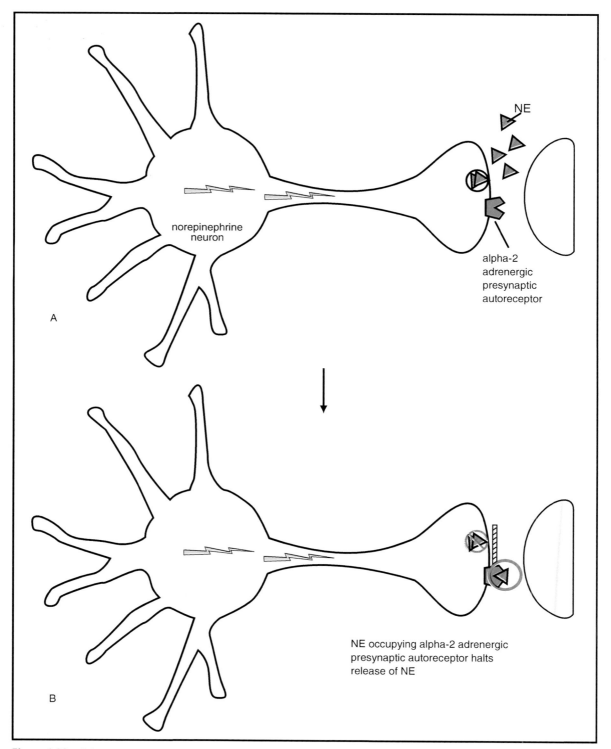

Figure 6-28. Alpha-2 receptors on axon terminal. Shown here are presynaptic α_2-adrenergic autoreceptors located on the axon terminal of the norepinephrine neuron. These autoreceptors are "gatekeepers" for norepinephrine. That is, when they are not bound by norepinephrine, they are open, allowing norepinephrine release (A). However, when norepinephrine binds to the gatekeeping receptors, they close the molecular gate and prevent norepinephrine from being released (B).

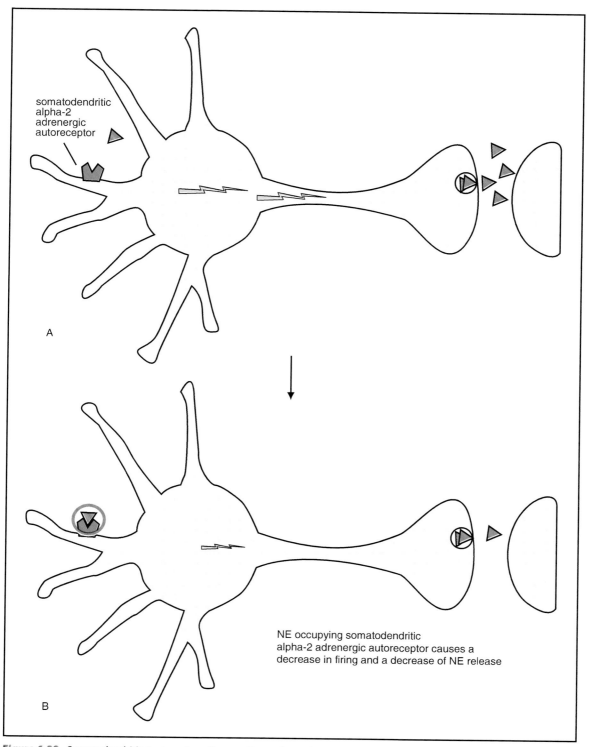

somatodendritic
alpha-2
adrenergic
autoreceptor

A

NE occupying somatodendritic
alpha-2 adrenergic autoreceptor causes a
decrease in firing and a decrease of NE release

B

Figure 6-29. **Somatodendritic α₂ receptors.** Presynaptic α₂-adrenergic autoreceptors are also located in the somatodendritic area of the norepinephrine neuron, as shown here. When norepinephrine binds to these α₂ receptors, it shuts off neuronal impulse flow in the norepinephrine neuron (see loss of lightning bolts in the neuron in the lower figure), and this stops further norepinephrine release.

same receptor will have the effect of cutting the brake cable, thus enhancing release of NE.

Monoamine interactions: NE regulation of 5HT release

Norepinephrine clearly regulates norepinephrine neurons via α_2 receptors (Figures 6-28 and 6-29); in Chapter 4, we showed that dopamine regulates dopamine neurons via D_2 receptors (Figures 4-8 through 4-10); and in Chapter 5 we showed that serotonin regulates serotonin neurons via $5HT_{1A}$ and $5HT_{1B/D}$ presynaptic receptors (Figures 5-25 and 5-27) and via $5HT_3$ receptors (illustrated in Chapter 7) and $5HT_7$ postsynaptic receptors (Figures 5-60A through 5-60C). Obviously, the three monoamines are all able to regulate their own release.

There are also numerous ways in which these three monoamines interact to regulate each other. For example, in Chapter 5 we showed that serotonin regulates dopamine release via $5HT_{1A}$ receptors (Figures 5-15C and 5-16C), $5HT_{2A}$ receptors (Figures 5-15A, 5-16A, 5-17) and $5HT_{2C}$ receptors (Figure 5-52A); we also showed that serotonin regulates norepinephrine release via $5HT_{2C}$ receptors (Figure 5-52A) and mentioned that serotonin regulates dopamine and norepinephrine via $5HT_3$ receptors, which is illustrated in Chapter 7 on antidepressants.

We now show that NE reciprocally regulates 5HT neurons via both α_1 and α_2 receptors (Figures 6-30A through 6-30C): α_1 receptors are the accelerator (Figure 6-30B), and α_2 receptors the brake (Figure 6-30C) on 5HT release. That is, NE neurons from the locus coeruleus travel a short distance to the midbrain raphe (Figure 6-30B, box 2) and there they release NE onto postsynaptic α_1 receptors on 5HT neuronal cell bodies. That directly stimulates 5HT neurons and acts as an accelerator for 5HT release, causing release of 5HT from their downstream axons (Figure 6-30B, box 1). Norepinephrine neurons also innervate the axon terminals of 5HT neurons (Figure 6-30C). Here NE is released directly onto postsynaptic α_2 receptors that inhibit 5HT neurons, acting as a brake on 5HT, thus inhibiting 5HT release (Figure 6-30C, box 1). Which action of NE predominates will depend upon which end of the 5HT neuron receives more noradrenergic input at any given time.

There are many brain areas where 5HT, NE, and DA projections overlap, creating opportunities for monoamine interactions throughout the brain and at many different receptor subtypes (Figures 6-31 through 6-33).

Numerous known inter-regulatory pathways and receptor interactions exist among the three monoaminergic neurotransmitter systems in order for them to influence each other and change the release not only of their own neurotransmitters, but also of other monoamines.

The monoamine hypothesis of depression

The classic theory about the biological etiology of depression hypothesizes that depression is due to a deficiency of monoamine neurotransmitters. Mania may be the opposite, due to an excess of monoamine neurotransmitters. At first, there was a great argument about whether norepinephrine (NE) or serotonin (5-hydroxytryptamine, 5HT) was the more important deficiency, and dopamine was relatively neglected. Now the monoamine theory suggests that the entire monoaminergic neurotransmitter system of all three monoamines NE, 5HT, and DA may be malfunctioning in various brain circuits, with different neurotransmitters involved depending upon the symptom profile of the patient.

The original conceptualization was rather simplistic and based upon observations that certain drugs that depleted these neurotransmitters could induce depression, and that all effective antidepressants act by boosting one or more of these three monoamine neurotransmitters. Thus, the idea was that the "normal" amount of monoamine neurotransmitters (Figure 6-34A) somehow became depleted, perhaps by an unknown disease process, by stress, or by drugs (Figure 6-34B), leading to the symptoms of depression.

Direct evidence for the monoamine hypothesis is still largely lacking. A good deal of effort was expended especially in the 1960s and 1970s to identify the theoretically predicted deficiencies of the monoamine neurotransmitters in depression and an excess in mania. This effort to date has unfortunately yielded mixed and sometimes confusing results, causing a search for better explanations of the potential link between monoamines and mood disorders.

The monoamine receptor hypothesis and gene expression

Because of these and other difficulties with the monoamine hypothesis, the focus of hypotheses for the etiology of mood disorders has shifted from the monoamine neurotransmitters themselves to their receptors

**Raphe Alpha 1 Receptors and Cortical Alpha 2 Receptors
Mediate Norepinephrine Regulation of 5HT Release**

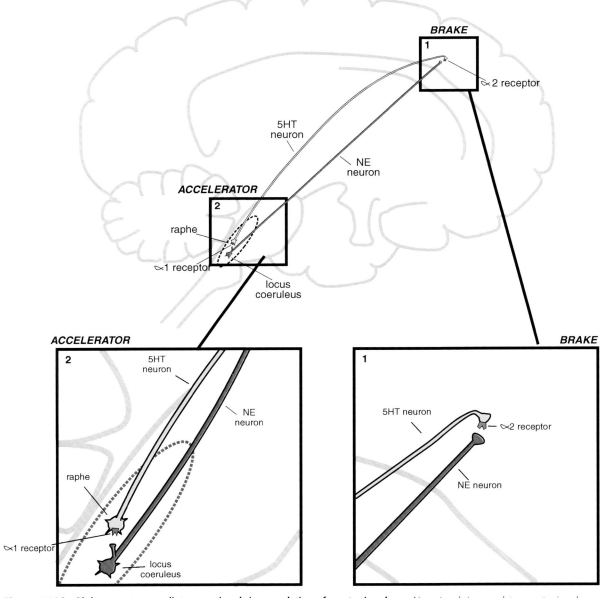

Figure 6-30A. Alpha receptors mediate norepinephrine regulation of serotonin release. Norepinephrine regulates serotonin release. It does this by acting as a brake on serotonin release at cortical a_2 receptors on axon terminals (1) and as an accelerator of serotonin release at a_1 receptors at the somatodendritic area (2).

Raphe Alpha 1 Receptors Stimulate Serotonin Release

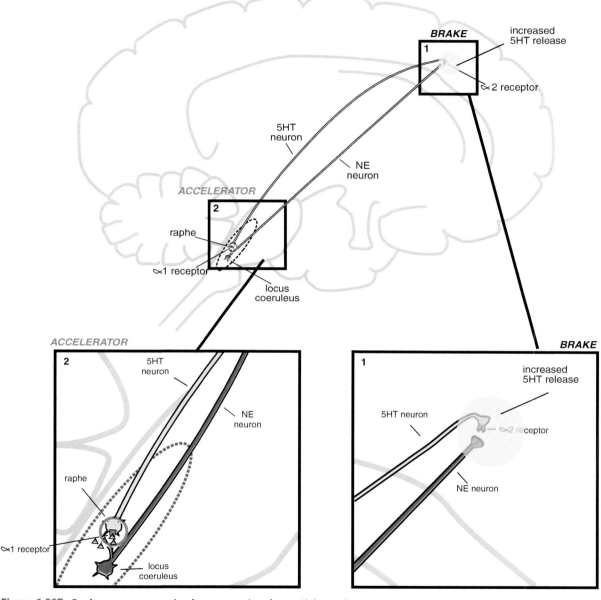

Figure 6-30B. Raphe α₁ receptors stimulate serotonin release. Alpha-1-adrenergic receptors are located in the somatodendritic regions of serotonin neurons. When these receptors are unoccupied by norepinephrine, some serotonin is released from the serotonin neuron. However, when norepinephrine binds to the α₁ receptor (2), this stimulates the serotonin neuron, accelerating release of serotonin (1).

Cortical Alpha 2 Receptors Inhibit Serotonin Release

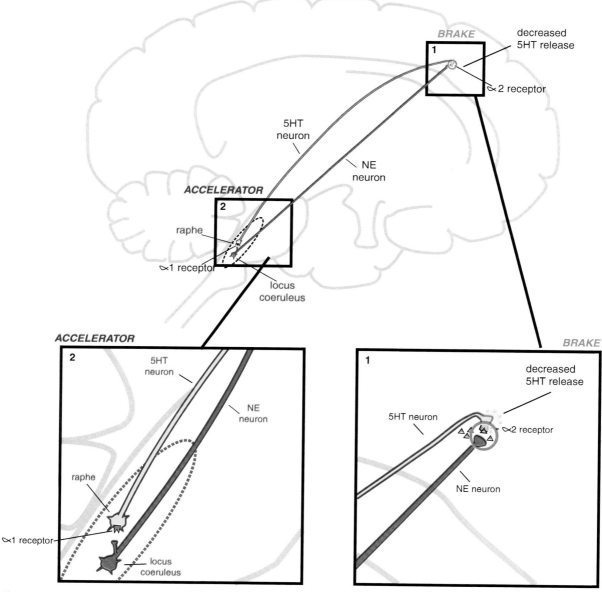

Figure 6-30C. Cortical α₂ receptors inhibit serotonin release. Alpha-2-adrenergic heteroreceptors are located on the axon terminals of serotonin neurons. When norepinephrine binds to the α₂ receptor this prevents serotonin from being released (1).

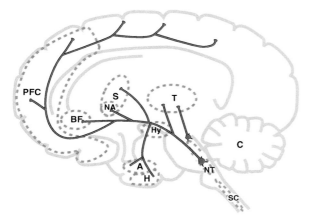

Figure 6-31. Major dopamine projections. Dopamine has widespread ascending projections that originate predominantly in the brainstem (particularly the ventral tegmental area and substantia nigra) and extend via the hypothalamus to the prefrontal cortex, basal forebrain, striatum, nucleus accumbens, and other regions. Dopaminergic neurotransmission is associated with movement, pleasure and reward, cognition, psychosis, and other functions. In addition, there are direct projections from other sites to the thalamus, creating the "thalamic dopamine system," which may be involved in arousal and sleep. PFC, prefrontal cortex; BF, basal forebrain; S, striatum; NA, nucleus accumbens; T, thalamus; Hy, hypothalamus; A, amygdala; H, hippocampus; NT, brainstem neurotransmitter centers; SC, spinal cord; C, cerebellum.

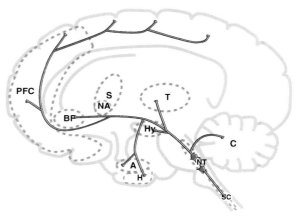

Figure 6-32. Major norepinephrine projections. Norepinephrine has both ascending and descending projections. Ascending noradrenergic projections originate mainly in the locus coeruleus of the brainstem; they extend to multiple brain regions, as shown here, and regulate mood, arousal, cognition, and other functions. Descending noradrenergic projections extend down the spinal cord and regulate pain pathways. PFC, prefrontal cortex; BF, basal forebrain; S, striatum; NA, nucleus accumbens; T, thalamus; Hy, hypothalamus; A, amygdala; H, hippocampus; NT, brainstem neurotransmitter centers; SC, spinal cord; C, cerebellum.

and the downstream molecular events that these receptors trigger, including the regulation of gene expression and the role of growth factors. There is also great interest in the influence of nature and nurture on brain circuits regulated by monoamines, especially what happens when epigenetic changes from stressful life experiences are combined with the inheritance of various risk genes that can make an individual vulnerable to those environmental stressors.

The neurotransmitter receptor hypothesis of depression posits that an abnormality in the receptors for monoamine neurotransmitters leads to depression (Figure 6-35). Thus, if depletion of monoamine neurotransmitters is the central theme of the monoamine hypothesis of depression (Figure 6-34B), the neurotransmitter receptor hypothesis of depression takes this theme one step further: namely, that the depletion of neurotransmitter causes compensatory upregulation of postsynaptic neurotransmitter receptors (Figure 6-35). Direct evidence for this hypothesis is also generally lacking. Postmortem studies do consistently show increased numbers of serotonin 2 receptors in the frontal cortex of patients who commit suicide. Also, some neuroimaging studies have identified abnormalities in serotonin receptors of depressed patients, but this approach has not yet been successful in identifying consistent and replicable molecular lesions in receptors

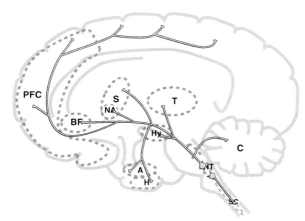

Figure 6-33. Major serotonin projections. Like norepinephrine, serotonin has both ascending and descending projections. Ascending serotonergic projections originate in the brainstem and extend to many of the same regions as noradrenergic projections, with additional projections to the striatum and nucleus accumbens. These ascending projections may regulate mood, anxiety, sleep, and other functions. Descending serotonergic projections extend down the brainstem and through the spinal cord; they may regulate pain. PFC, prefrontal cortex; BF, basal forebrain; S, striatum; NA, nucleus accumbens; T, thalamus; Hy, hypothalamus; A, amygdala; H, hippocampus; NT, brainstem neurotransmitter centers; SC, spinal cord; C, cerebellum.

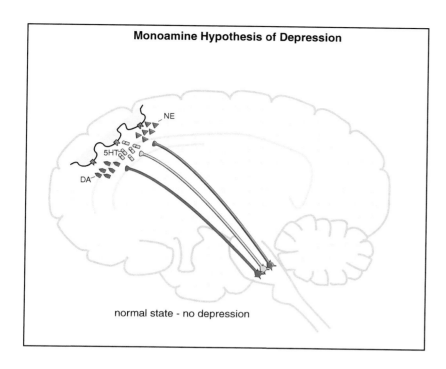

Figure 6-34A. Classic monoamine hypothesis of depression, part 1. According to the classic monoamine hypothesis of depression, when there is a "normal" amount of monoamine neurotransmitter activity, there is no depression present.

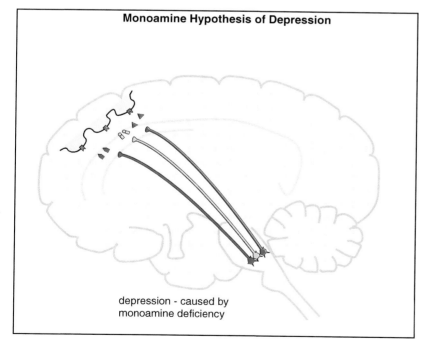

Figure 6-34B. Classic monoamine hypothesis of depression, part 2. The monoamine hypothesis of depression posits that if the "normal" amount of monoamine neurotransmitter activity becomes reduced, depleted, or dysfunctional for some reason, depression may ensue.

for monoamines in depression. Thus, there is no clear and convincing evidence that monoamine deficiency accounts for depression – i.e., there is no "real" monoamine deficit. Likewise, there is no clear and convincing evidence that abnormalities in monoamine receptors account for depression. Although the monoamine hypothesis is obviously an overly simplified notion about mood disorders, it has been very valuable in

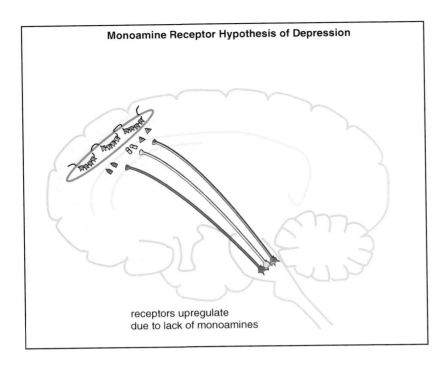

Monoamine Receptor Hypothesis of Depression

receptors upregulate
due to lack of monoamines

Figure 6-35. Monoamine receptor hypothesis of depression. The monoamine receptor hypothesis of depression extends the classic monoamine hypothesis of depression, positing that deficient activity of monoamine neurotransmitters causes upregulation of postsynaptic monoamine neurotransmitter receptors, and that this leads to depression.

focusing attention upon the three monoamine neurotransmitter systems norepinephrine, dopamine, and serotonin. This has led to a much better understanding of the physiological functioning of these three neurotransmitters, and especially the various mechanisms by which all known antidepressants act to boost neurotransmission at one or more of these three monoamine neurotransmitter systems, and how certain mood-stabilizing drugs may also act on the monoamines. Research is now turning to the possibility that in depression there may be a deficiency in downstream signal transduction of the monoamine neurotransmitter and its postsynaptic neuron that is occurring in the presence of normal amounts of neurotransmitter and receptor. Thus, the hypothesized molecular problem in depression could lie within the molecular events distal to the receptor, in the signal transduction cascade system, and in appropriate gene expression (Figure 6-36). Different molecular problems may account for mania and bipolar disorder.

Stress and depression

Stress, BDNF, and brain atrophy in depression

One candidate mechanism that has been proposed as the site of a possible flaw in signal transduction from monoamine receptors in depression is the target gene for brain-derived neurotrophic factor (BDNF) (Figures 6-36, 6-37, 6-38). Normally, BDNF sustains the viability of brain neurons (Figure 6-37), but under stress, the gene for BDNF may be repressed (Figure 6-38). Stress can lower 5HT levels and can acutely increase, then chronically deplete, both NE and DA. These monoamine neurotransmitter changes together with deficient amounts of BDNF may lead to atrophy and possible apoptosis of vulnerable neurons in the hippocampus and other brain areas such as prefrontal cortex (Figure 6-37). An artist's concept of the hippocampal atrophy that has been reported in association with chronic stress and with both major depression and various anxiety disorders, especially PTSD, is shown in Figures 6-39A and 6-39B. Fortunately, some of this neuronal loss may be reversible. That is, restoration of monoamine-related signal transduction cascades by antidepressants (Figure 6-36) can increase BDNF and other trophic factors (Figure 6-37) and potentially restore lost synapses. In some brain areas such as the hippocampus, not only can synapses potentially be restored, but it is possible that some lost neurons might even be replaced by neurogenesis.

Neurons from the hippocampal area and amygdala normally suppress the hypothalamic–pituitary–adrenal (HPA) axis (Figure 6-39A), so if stress causes hippocampal and amygdala neurons to atrophy, with loss of

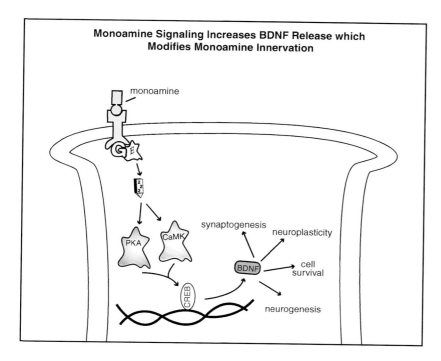

Monoamine Signaling Increases BDNF Release which
Modifies Monoamine Innervation

monoamine

synaptogenesis
neuroplasticity

PKA   CaMK

BDNF   cell
survival

CREB

neurogenesis

Figure 6-36. Monoamine signaling and brain-derived neurotrophic factor (BDNF) release. The neurotrophic hypothesis of depression states that depression may be caused by reduced synthesis of proteins involved in neurogenesis and synaptic plasticity. BDNF promotes the growth and development of immature neurons, including monoaminergic neurons, enhances the survival and function of adult neurons, and helps maintain synaptic connections. Because BDNF is important for neuronal survival, decreased levels may contribute to cell atrophy. In some cases, low levels of BDNF may even cause cell loss. Monoamines can increase the availability of BDNF by initiating signal transduction cascades that lead to its release. Thus, if monoamine levels are low, then BDNF levels may correspondingly be low. CaMK, calcium/calmodulin-dependent protein kinase; CREB, cAMP response element-binding protein; PKA, protein kinase A.

their inhibitory input to the hypothalamus, this could lead to overactivity of the HPA axis (Figure 6-39B). In depression, abnormalities of the HPA axis have long been reported, including elevated glucocorticoid levels and insensitivity of the HPA axis to feedback inhibition (Figure 6-39B). Some evidence suggests that glucocorticoids at high levels could even be toxic to neurons and contribute to their atrophy under chronic stress (Figure 6-39B). Novel antidepressant treatments are in testing that target corticotropin-releasing factor 1 (CRF-1) receptors, vasopressin 1B receptors, and glucocorticoid receptors (Figure 6-39B), in an attempt to halt and even reverse these HPA abnormalities in depression and other stress-related psychiatric illnesses.

Stress and the environment: how much stress is too much stress?

In many ways the body is built for the purpose of handling stress, and in fact a certain amount of "stress load" on bones, muscles, and brain is necessary for growth and optimal functioning and can even be associated with developing resilience to future stressors (Figure 6-40). However, certain types of stress such as child abuse can sensitize brain circuits and render them vulnerable rather than resilient to future stressors (Figure 6-41).

For patients with such vulnerable brain circuits who then become exposed to multiple life stressors as adults, the result can be the development of depression (Figure 6-42). Thus, the same amount of stress that would be handled without developing depression in someone who has not experienced child abuse could hypothetically cause depression in someone with a prior history of child abuse. This demonstrates the potential impact of the environment upon brain circuits. Many studies in fact confirm that in women abused as children, depression can be found up to four times more often than in never-abused women. Hypothetically, epigenetic changes caused by environmental stress create relatively permanent molecular alterations in the brain circuits at the time of the child abuse that do not cause depression per se, but make brain circuits vulnerable to breakdown into depression upon exposure to future stressors as an adult.

Stress and vulnerability genes: born fearful?

Modern theories of mood disorders do not propose that any single gene can cause depression or mania, but as discussed for schizophrenia in Chapter 4

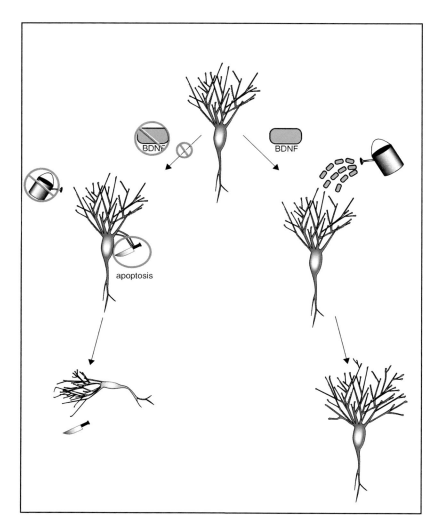

Figure 6-37. Suppression of brain-derived neurotrophic factor (BDNF) production. BDNF plays a role in the proper growth and maintenance of neurons and neuronal connections (right). If the genes for BDNF are turned off (left), the resultant decrease in BDNF could compromise the brain's ability to create and maintain neurons and their connections. This could lead to loss of synapses or even whole neurons by apoptosis.

(see also Figure 4-33), mood disorders are theoretically caused by a "conspiracy" among many vulnerability genes and many environmental stressors leading to breakdown of information processing in specific brain circuits and thus the various symptoms of a major depressive or manic episode. There is a great overlap between those genes thought to be vulnerability genes for schizophrenia and those thought to be vulnerability genes for bipolar disorder. A comprehensive discussion of genes for bipolar disorder or for major depression is beyond the scope of this book, but one of the vulnerability genes for depression is the gene coding for the serotonin transporter or SERT (i.e., the serotonin reuptake pump), which is the site of action of SSRI and SNRI antidepressants. The type of serotonin transporter (SERT)

with which you are born determines in part whether your amygdala is more likely to over-react to fearful faces (Figure 6-43), whether you are more likely to develop depression when exposed to multiple life stressors, and how likely your depression is to respond to an SSRI/SNRI or whether you can even tolerate an SSRI/SNRI (Figure 6-43).

Specifically, an excessive reaction of the amygdala to fearful faces for carriers of the s variant of the gene for SERT is shown in Figure 6-43. Fearful faces can be considered a stressful load on the amygdala and its circuitry, and can be visualized using modern neuroimaging techniques. For those with the s genotype of SERT, they are more likely to develop an affective disorder when exposed to multiple life stressors and may have more hippocampal

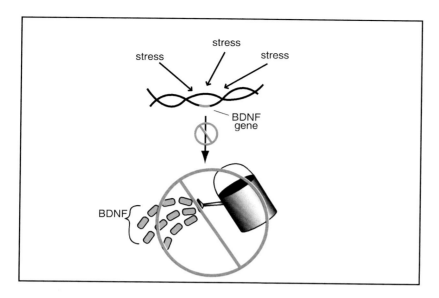

Figure 6-38. Stress and brain-derived neurotrophic factor (BDNF). One factor that could contribute to potential brain atrophy is the impact that chronic stress can have on BDNF, which plays a role in the proper growth and maintenance of neurons and neuronal connections. During chronic stress, the genes for BDNF may be turned off, potentially reducing its production.

The Hypothalamic - Pituitary - Adrenal (HPA) Axis

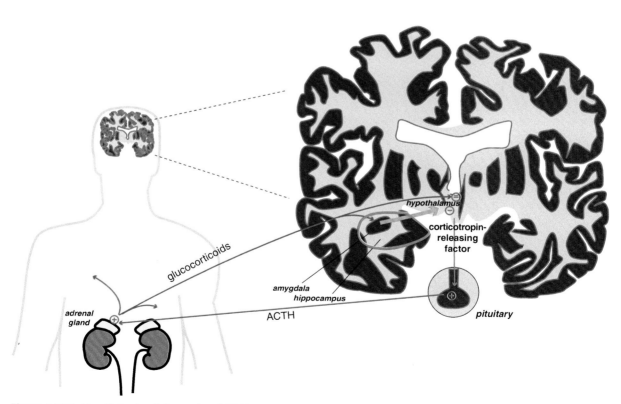

Figure 6-39A. Hypothalamic–pituitary–adrenal (HPA) axis. The normal stress response involves activation of the hypothalamus and a resultant increase in corticotropin-releasing factor (CRF), which in turn stimulates the release of adrenocorticotropic hormone (ACTH) from the pituitary. ACTH causes glucocorticoid release from the adrenal gland, which feeds back to the hypothalamus and inhibits CRF release, terminating the stress response.

Hippocampal Atrophy and Hyperactive HPA in Depression

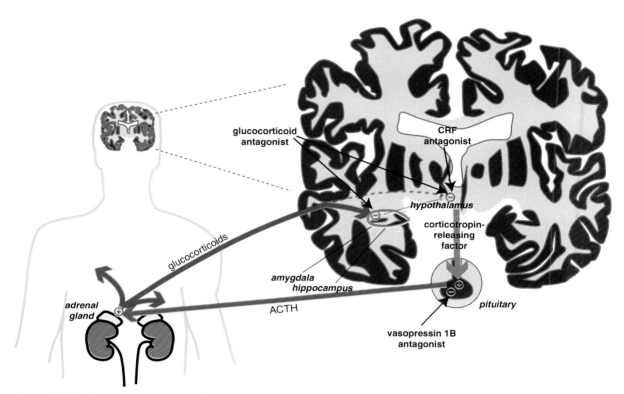

Figure 6-39B. **Hippocampal atrophy and hyperactive HPA axis in depression.** In situations of chronic stress, excessive glucocorticoid release may eventually cause hippocampal atrophy. Because the hippocampus inhibits the HPA axis, atrophy in this region may lead to chronic activation of the HPA axis, which may increase risk of developing a psychiatric illness. Because the HPA axis is central to stress processing, it may be that novel targets for treating stress-induced disorders lie within the axis. Mechanisms being examined include antagonism of glucocorticoid receptors, corticotropin-releasing factor 1 (CRF-1) receptors, and vasopressin 1B receptors.

atrophy, more cognitive symptoms, and less responsiveness or tolerance to SSRI/SNRI treatment. Exposure to multiple life stressors may cause the otherwise silent overactivity and inefficient information processing of affective loads in the amygdala to become an overt major depressive episode (Figure 6-43), an interaction of their genes with the environment (nature plus nurture). The point is that the specific gene that you have for the serotonin transporter can alter the efficiency of affective information processing by your amygdala and, consequently, your risk for developing major depression if you experience multiple life stressors as an adult (Figure 6-43). On the other hand, the l genotype of SERT is a more resilient genotype, with less amygdala reactivity to fearful faces, less likelihood of breaking down into a major depressive episode when exposed to multiple life stressors, as well as more likelihood of responding to or tolerating SSRIs/SNRIs if you do develop a depressive episode (Figure 6-43).

Whether you have the l or the s genotype of SERT accounts for only a small amount of the variance for whether or not you will develop major depression after experiencing multiple life stressors, and thus cannot predict who will get major depression and who will not. However, this example does prove the importance of genes in general and those for serotonin neurons in particular in the regulation of the amygdala and in determining the odds of developing major depression under stress. Thus, perhaps one is not born fearful, but born vulnerable or resilient to

Development of Stress Resilience

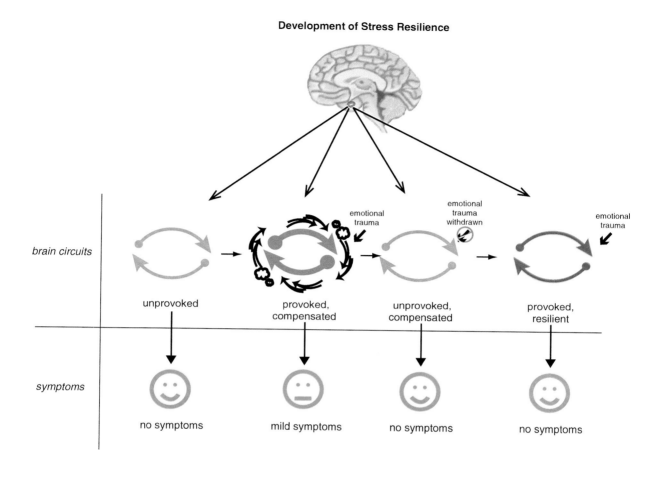

brain circuits

- unprovoked
- provoked, compensated
- unprovoked, compensated
- provoked, resilient

emotional trauma

emotional trauma withdrawn

emotional trauma

symptoms

- no symptoms
- mild symptoms
- no symptoms
- no symptoms

overactivation
normal
baseline
hypoactivation

Figure 6-40. Development of stress resilience. In a healthy individual, stress can cause a temporary activation of circuits which is resolved when the stressor is removed. As shown here, when the circuit is unprovoked, no symptoms are produced. In the presence of a stressor such as emotional trauma, the circuit is provoked yet able to compensate for the effects of the stressor. By its ability to process the information load from the environment, it can avoid producing symptoms. When the stressor is withdrawn, the circuit returns to baseline functioning. Individuals exposed to this type of short-term stress may even develop resilience to stress, whereby exposure to future stressors provokes the circuit but does not result in symptoms.

developing major depression in response to future adult stressors, especially if they are chronic, multiple, and severe.

Symptoms and circuits in depression

Currently, the monoamine hypothesis of depression is now being applied to understanding how monoamines regulate the efficiency of information processing in a wide variety of neuronal circuits that may be responsible for mediating the various symptoms of depression. Obviously, there are numerous symptoms required for the diagnosis of a major depressive episode (Figure 6-44). Each symptom is hypothetically associated with inefficient information processing in various brain circuits, with different symptoms topographically localized to specific brain regions (Figure 6-45).

Development of Stress Sensitization

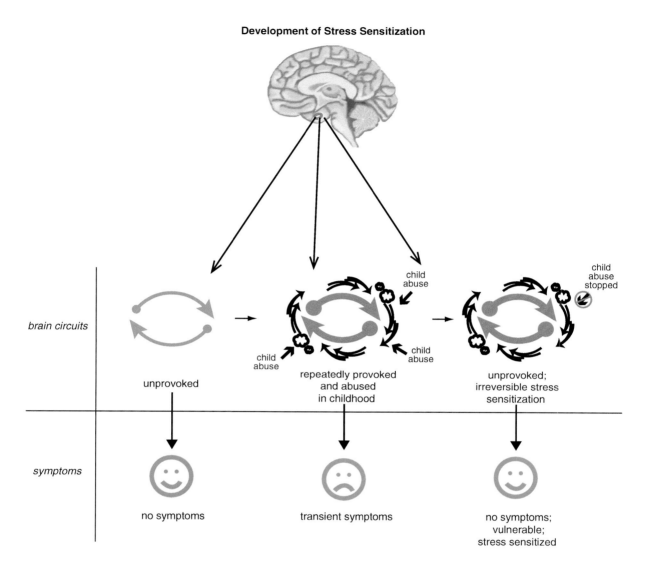

brain circuits

unprovoked

child abuse

child abuse

repeatedly provoked and abused in childhood

child abuse

child abuse stopped

unprovoked; irreversible stress sensitization

symptoms

no symptoms

transient symptoms

no symptoms; vulnerable; stress sensitized

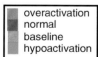

overactivation
normal
baseline
hypoactivation

Figure 6-41. Development of stress sensitization. Prolonged activation of circuits due to repeated exposure to stressors can lead to a condition known as "stress sensitization," in which circuits not only become overly activated but remain overly activated even when the stressor is withdrawn. Thus, an individual with severe stress in childhood will exhibit transient symptoms during stress exposure, with resolution of the symptoms when the stressor is removed. The circuits remain overly activated in this model, but the individual exhibits no symptoms because these circuits can somehow still compensate for this additional load. However, the individual with "stress-sensitized" circuits is now vulnerable to the effects of future stressors, so that the risk for developing psychiatric symptoms is increased. Stress sensitization may therefore constitute a "presymptomatic" state for some psychiatric symptoms. This state might be detectable with functional brain scans of circuits but not from psychiatric interviews or patient complaints.

Progression from Stress Sensitization to Depression

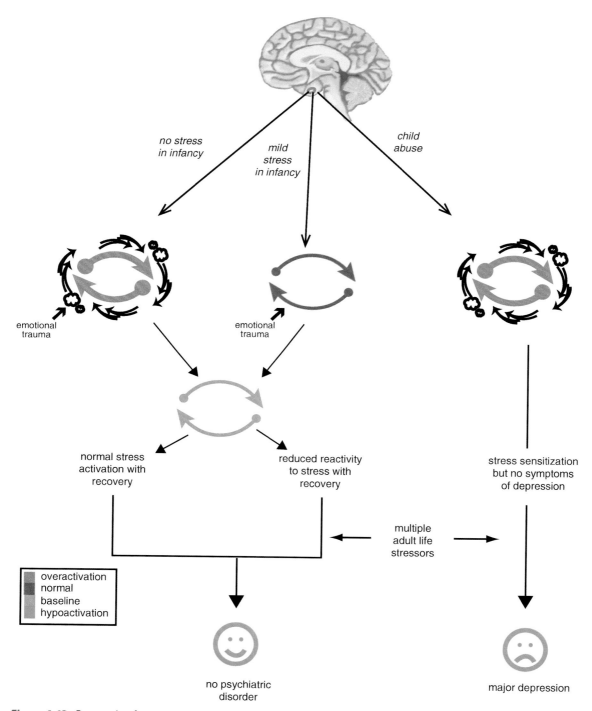

Figure 6-42. Progression from stress sensitization to depression. It may be that the degree of stress one experiences during early life affects how the circuits develop and therefore how a given individual responds to stress in later life. No stress during infancy may lead to a circuit that exhibits "normal" activation during stress and confers no increased risk of developing a psychiatric disorder. Interestingly, mild stress during infancy may actually cause the circuits to exhibit reduced reactivity to stress in later life and provide some resilience to adult stressors. Overwhelming and/or chronic stress from child abuse, however, may lead to stress-sensitized circuits that may become activated even in the absence of a stressor. Individuals with stress sensitization may not exhibit phenotypic symptoms but may be at increased risk of developing a mental illness if exposed to future stressors.

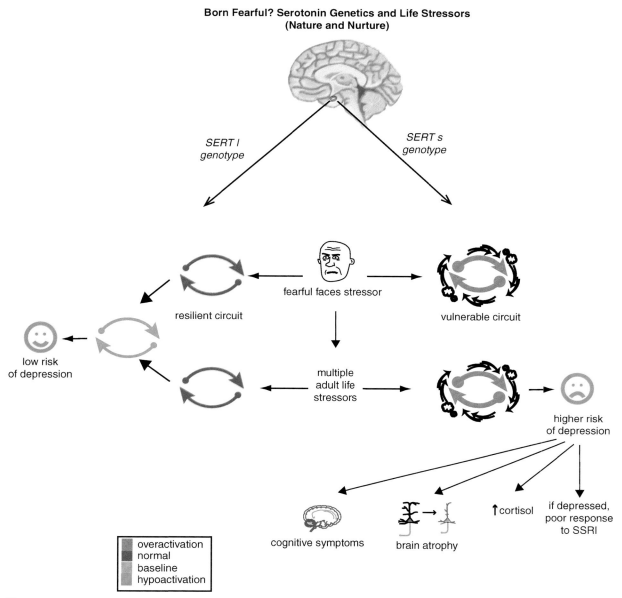

Born Fearful? Serotonin Genetics and Life Stressors (Nature and Nurture)

SERT l genotype

SERT s genotype

fearful faces stressor

resilient circuit

vulnerable circuit

low risk of depression

multiple adult life stressors

higher risk of depression

overactivation
normal
baseline
hypoactivation

cognitive symptoms

brain atrophy

↑ cortisol

if depressed, poor response to SSRI

Figure 6-43. **Serotonin genetics and life stressors.** Genetic research has shown that the type of serotonin transporter (SERT) with which you are born can affect how you process fearful stimuli and perhaps also how you respond to stress. Specifically, individuals who are carriers of the s variant of the gene for SERT appear to be more vulnerable to the effects of stress or anxiety, whereas those who carry the l variant appear to be more resilient. Thus, s carriers exhibit increased amygdala activity in response to fearful faces and may also be more likely to develop a mood or anxiety disorder after suffering multiple life stressors. The higher risk of depression may also be related to increased likelihood of cognitive symptoms, brain atrophy, increased cortisol, and, if depressed, poor response to selective serotonin reuptake inhibitors (SSRIs).

Not only can each of the nine symptoms listed for the diagnosis of a major depressive episode be mapped onto brain circuits whose inefficient information processing theoretically mediates these symptoms (Figure 6-45), but the hypothetical monoaminergic regulation of each of these various brain areas can also be mapped onto each brain region they innervate (Figures 6-31 through 6-33). This creates a set of monoamine neurotransmitters that regulates each specific hypothetically malfunctioning brain region. Targeting each region with

Symptom Dimensions of a Major Depressive Episode

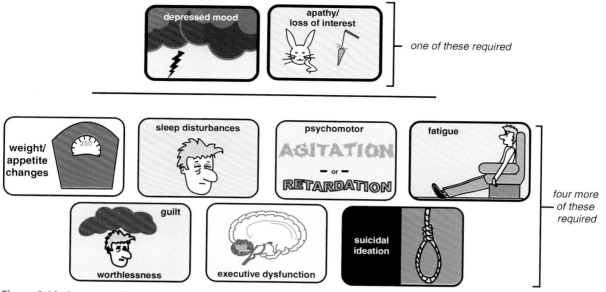

Figure 6-44. Symptoms of depression. According to the *Diagnostic and Statistical Manual of Mental Disorders*, a major depressive episode consists of either depressed mood or loss of interest and at least four of the following: weight/appetite changes, insomnia or hypersomnia, psychomotor agitation or retardation, fatigue, feelings of guilt or worthlessness, executive dysfunction, and suicidal ideation.

Match Each Diagnostic Symptom for a Major Depressive Episode to Hypothetically Malfunctioning Brain Circuits

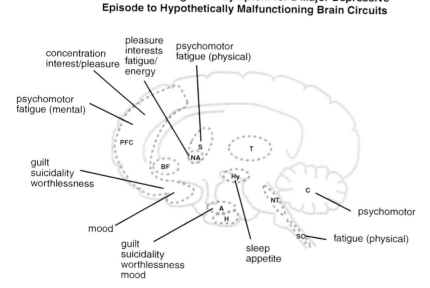

Figure 6-45. Matching depression symptoms to circuits. Alterations in neuronal activity and in the efficiency of information processing within each of the eleven brain regions shown here can lead to symptoms of a major depressive episode. Functionality in each brain region is hypothetically associated with a different constellation of symptoms. PFC, prefrontal cortex; BF, basal forebrain; S, striatum; NA, nucleus accumbens; T, thalamus; Hy, hypothalamus; A, amygdala; H, hippocampus; NT, brainstem neurotransmitter centers; SC, spinal cord; C, cerebellum.

drugs that act on the relevant monoamine(s) that innervate those brain regions potentially leads to reduction of each individual symptom experienced by a specific patient by enhancing the efficiency of information processing in malfunctioning circuits for each specific symptom. If successful, this targeting of monoamines in specific brain areas could even eliminate symptoms, and cause a major depressive episode to go into remission.

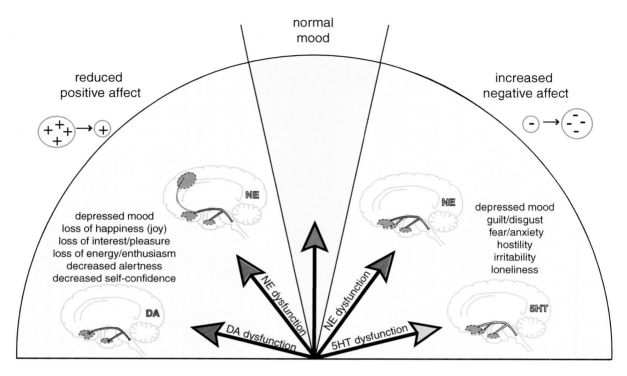

Figure 6-46. Positive and negative affect. Mood-related symptoms of depression can be characterized by their affective expression – that is, whether they cause a reduction in positive affect or an increase in negative affect. Symptoms related to reduced positive affect include depressed mood; loss of happiness, interest, or pleasure; loss of energy or enthusiasm; decreased alertness; and decreased self-confidence. Reduced positive affect may be hypothetically related to dopaminergic dysfunction, with a possible role of noradrenergic dysfunction as well. Symptoms associated with increased negative affect include depressed mood, guilt, disgust, fear, anxiety, hostility, irritability, and loneliness. Increased negative affect may be linked hypothetically to serotonergic dysfunction and perhaps also noradrenergic dysfunction.

Many of the mood-related symptoms of depression can be categorized as having either too little positive affect, or too much negative affect (Figure 6-46). This idea is linked to the fact that there are diffuse anatomic connections of monoamines throughout the brain, with diffuse dopamine dysfunction in this system driving predominantly the reduction of positive affect, diffuse serotonin dysfunction driving predominantly the increase in negative affect, and norepinephrine dysfunction being involved in both. Thus, reduced positive affect includes such symptoms as depressed mood but also loss of happiness, joy, interest, pleasure, alertness, energy, enthusiasm, and self-confidence (Figure 6-46, left). Enhancing dopamine function, and possibly also norepinephrine function may improve information processing in the circuits mediating this cluster of symptoms. On the other hand, increased negative affect includes not only depressed mood but guilt, disgust, fear, anxiety, hostility, irritability and loneliness (Figure 6-46, right). Enhancing serotonin function, and possibly also

norepinephrine function, may improve information processing in the circuits that hypothetically mediate this cluster of symptoms. For patients with symptoms of both clusters, they may require triple-action treatments that boost all three of the monoamines.

Symptoms and circuits in mania

The same general paradigm of monoamine regulation of the efficiency of information processing in specific brain circuits can be applied to mania as well as depression, although this is frequently thought to be in the opposite direction and in some overlapping but also some different brain regions compared to depression. The numerous symptoms required for the diagnosis of a manic episode are shown in Figure 6-47. Like major depression, each symptom of mania is also hypothetically associated with inefficient information processing in various brain circuits, with different symptoms topographically localized to specific brain regions (Figure 6-48).

Symptom Dimensions of a Manic Episode

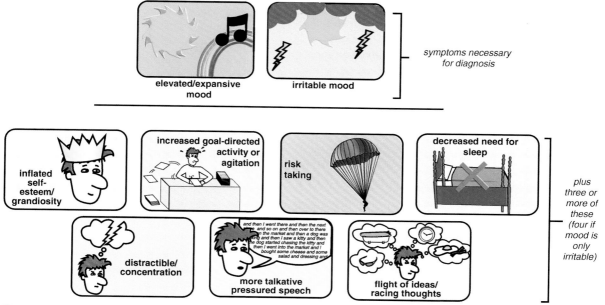

Figure 6-47. Symptoms of mania. According to the *Diagnostic and Statistical Manual of Mental Disorders*, a manic episode consists of either elevated/expansive mood or irritable mood. In addition, at least three of the following must be present (four if mood is irritable): inflated self-esteem/grandiosity, increased goal-directed activity or agitation, risk taking, decreased need for sleep, distractibility, pressured speech, and racing thoughts.

Match Each Diagnostic Symptom for a Manic Episode to Hypothetically Malfunctioning Brain Circuits

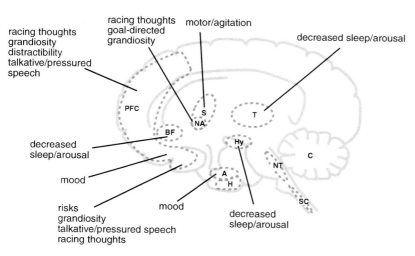

Figure 6-48. Matching mania symptoms to circuits. Alterations in neurotransmission within each of the eleven brain regions shown here can be hypothetically linked to the various symptoms of a manic episode. Functionality in each brain region may be associated with a different constellation of symptoms. PFC, prefrontal cortex; BF, basal forebrain; S, striatum; NA, nucleus accumbens; T, thalamus; Hy, hypothalamus; A, amygdala; H, hippocampus; NT, brainstem neurotransmitter centers; SC, spinal cord; C, cerebellum.

Generally, the inefficient functioning in these circuits in mania may be essentially the opposite of the malfunctioning hypothesized for depression, but may be more accurately portrayed as "out of tune" rather than simply excessive or deficient, especially since some patients can simultaneously have both manic and depressed symptoms. Generally, treatments for mania either reduce or stabilize monoaminergic regulation of circuits associated with symptoms of mania.

Neuroimaging in mood disorders

It is not currently possible to diagnose depression or bipolar disorder with any neuroimaging technique. However, some progress is being made in mapping inefficient information processing in various circuits in mood disorders. In depression, the dorsolateral prefrontal cortex, associated with cognitive symp- toms, may have reduced activity, and the amygdala, associated with various emotional symptoms includ- ing depressed mood, may have increased activity (Figure 6-49). Furthermore, provocative testing of patients with mood disorders may provide some insight into malfunctioning of brain circuits exposed to environmental input, and thus required to process that information. For example, some studies of

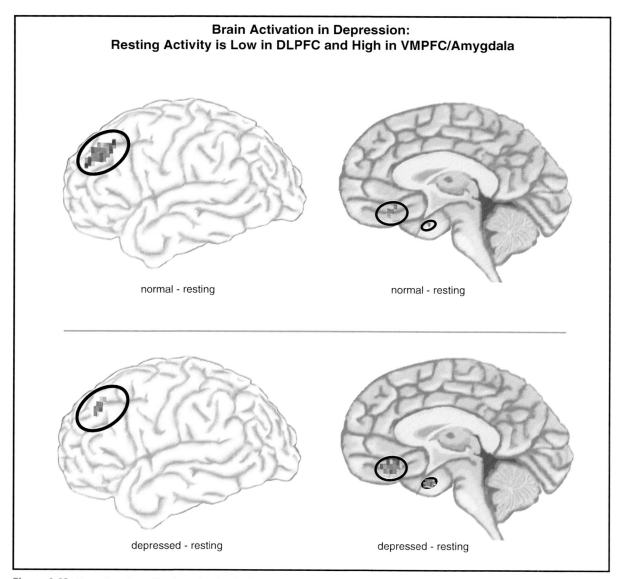

**Brain Activation in Depression:
Resting Activity is Low in DLPFC and High in VMPFC/Amygdala**

normal - resting

normal - resting

depressed - resting

depressed - resting

Figure 6-49. **Neuroimaging of brain activation in depression.** Neuroimaging studies of brain activation suggest that resting activity in the dorsolateral prefrontal cortex (DLPFC) of depressed patients is low compared to that in nondepressed individuals (left, top and bottom), whereas resting activity in the amygdala and ventromedial prefrontal cortex (VMPFC) of depressed patients is high compared to that in nondepressed individuals (right, top and bottom).

**Depressed Patients May Be More Responsive to
Induction of Sadness Than to Induction of Happiness**

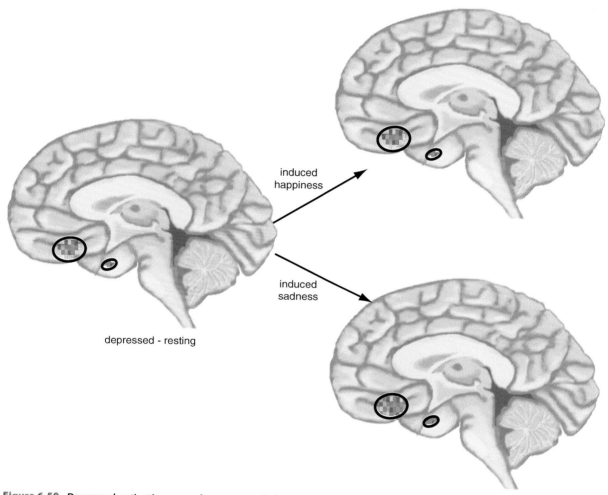

induced
happiness

induced
sadness

depressed - resting

Figure 6-50. Depressed patient's neuronal response to induced sadness versus happiness. Emotional symptoms such as sadness or happiness are regulated by the ventromedial prefrontal cortex (VMPFC) and the amygdala, two regions in which activity is high in the resting state of depressed patients (left). Interestingly, provocative tests in which these emotions are induced show that neuronal activity in the amygdala is over-reactive to induced sadness (bottom right) but under-reactive to induced happiness (top right).

depressed patients show that their neuronal circuits at the level of the amygdala are over-reactive to induced sadness but under-reactive to induced happiness (Figure 6-50). On the other hand, imaging of the orbitofrontal cortex of manic patients shows that they fail to appropriately activate this brain region in a test that requires them to suppress a response, suggesting problems with impulsivity associated with mania and with this specific brain region (Figure 6-51). In general, these neuroimaging findings support the mapping of symptoms to brain regions discussed earlier in this chapter, but much further work is currently in progress and must be completed before the results of neuroimaging can be applied to diagnostic or therapeutic decision making in clinical practice.

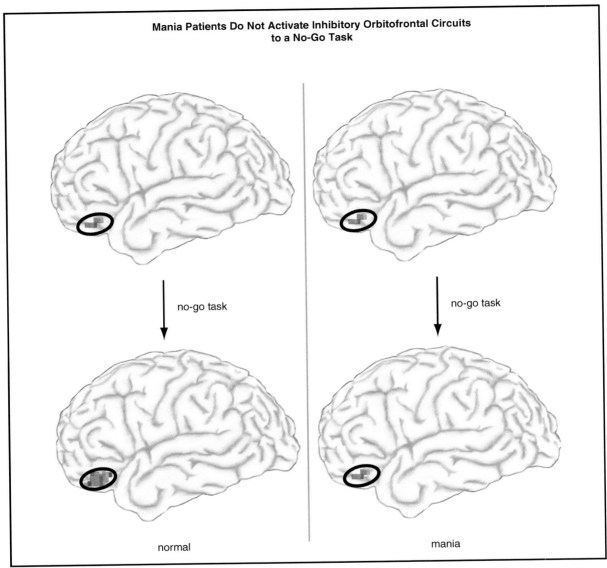

Mania Patients Do Not Activate Inhibitory Orbitofrontal Circuits to a No-Go Task

no-go task

no-go task

normal

mania

Figure 6-51. Mania patient's neuronal response to no-go task. Impulsive symptoms of mania, such as risk taking and pressured speech, are related to activity in the orbitofrontal cortex (OFC). Neuroimaging data show that this brain region is hypoactive in mania (bottom right) versus healthy (bottom left) individuals during the no-go task, which is designed to test response inhibition.

Summary

This chapter has described the mood disorders, including those across the bipolar spectrum. For prognostic and treatment purposes, it is increasingly important to be able to distinguish unipolar depression from bipolar spectrum depression. Although mood disorders are indeed disorders of mood, they are much more, and several different symptoms in addition to a mood symptom are required to make a diagnosis of a major depressive episode or a manic episode. Each symptom can be matched to a hypothetically malfunctioning neuronal circuit. The monoamine hypothesis of depression suggests that dysfunction, generally due to underactivity, of one or more of the three monoamines DA, NE, or 5HT may be linked to symptoms in major depression. Boosting one or more of the monoamines in specific brain regions may improve the efficiency of information processing there, and reduce the symptom caused by that area's malfunctioning. Other brain areas associated with the symptoms of a manic episode can similarly be mapped to various hypothetically malfunctioning brain circuits. Understanding the localization of symptoms in circuits, as well as the neurotransmitters that regulate these circuits in different brain regions, can set the stage for choosing and combining treatments for each individual symptom of a mood disorder, with the goal being to reduce all symptoms and lead to remission.

Chapter 7

Antidepressants

In this chapter, we will review pharmacological concepts underlying the use of antidepressant drugs. There are many different classes of antidepressants and dozens of individual drugs. The goal of this chapter is to acquaint the reader with current ideas about how the various antidepressants work. We will explain the mechanisms of action of these drugs by building upon general pharmacological concepts introduced in earlier chapters. We will also discuss concepts about how to use these drugs in clinical practice, including strategies for what to do if initial treatments fail and how to rationally combine one antidepressant with another, or with a modulating agent. Finally, we will introduce the reader to several new antidepressants in clinical development.

Our discussion of antidepressants in this chapter is at the conceptual level, and not at the pragmatic level. The reader should consult standard drug handbooks (such as the companion *Stahl's Essential Psychopharmacology: the Prescriber's Guide*) for details of doses, side effects, drug interactions, and other issues relevant to the prescribing of these drugs in clinical practice. Here we will discuss putting together an antidepressant "portfolio" of two or more mechanisms of action, often requiring more than one drug, as a strategy for patients who have not responded to a single pharmacological mechanism. This treatment strategy for depression is very different than that for schizophrenia, where single antipsychotic drugs as treatments are the rule and the expected improvement in symptomatology may be only a 20–30% reduction of symptoms with few if any patients with schizophrenia becoming truly asymptomatic and in remission. Thus, the chance to reach a genuine state of sustained and asymptomatic remission in major depression is the challenge for those who treat this disorder; this is the reason for learning the mechanisms of action of so many drugs, the complex biological rationale for combining specific sets of drugs, and the practical tactics for tailoring a unique drug treatment portfolio to fit the needs of an individual patient.

General principles of antidepressant action

Patients who have a major depressive episode and who receive treatment with any antidepressant often experience improvement in their symptoms, and when this improvement reaches the level of 50% reduction of symptoms or more, it is called a response (Figure 7-1). This used to be the goal of treatment with antidepressants: namely, reduce symptoms substantially, and at least by 50%. However, the paradigm for antidepressant treatment has shifted dramatically in recent years so that now the goal of treatment is complete remission of symptoms (Figure 7-2), while maintaining that level of improvement so that the patient's major depressive episode does not relapse shortly after remission, nor does the patient have a recurrent episode in the future (Figure 7-3). Given the known limits to the efficacy of available antidepressants, especially when multiple antidepressant treatment options are not deployed aggressively and early in the course of this illness, the goal of sustained remission can be difficult to reach. In fact, remission is usually not even reached with the first antidepressant treatment choice.

Do antidepressants work anymore in clinical trials?

Although remission (Figure 7-2) without relapse or recurrence (Figure 7-3) is the widely accepted goal of antidepressant treatment, it is becoming more and more difficult to prove that antidepressants – even well-established antidepressants – work any better than placebo in clinical trials. This is generally due to the fact that in modern clinical trials, the placebo effect has inflated so much over recent decades that placebo now seems to work as well as antidepressants in some trials and nearly as well as antidepressants in other trials. Why this is occurring is the subject of vigorous debate. Some experts propose that it is due to problems conducting clinical ratings in a clinical trial setting that is now unlike a clinical practice setting since patients are seen weekly, often for hours, whether they receive an antidepressant or not; other experts point out that subjects in trials may really be "symptomatic volunteers" who are less ill and less complicated than "real" patients. Critics of psychiatry and psychopharmacology proclaim from clinical trial evidence that antidepressants don't even work and that their side effects and costs do not justify their use at all. This phenomenon of shrinking and erratic efficacy of long-established antidepressants as well as new antidepressants in clinical trials has also caused

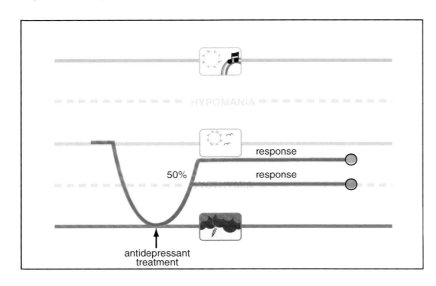

Figure 7-1. Response. When treatment of depression results in at least 50% improvement in symptoms, it is called a response. Such patients are better but not well. Previously, this was considered the goal of depression treatment.

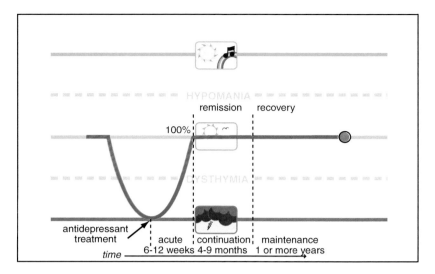

Figure 7-2. Remission. When treatment of depression results in removal of essentially all symptoms, it is called remission for the first several months and then recovery if it is sustained for longer than 6 months. Such patients are not just better – they are well. However, they are not cured, since depression can still recur. Remission and recovery are now the goals when treating patients with depression.

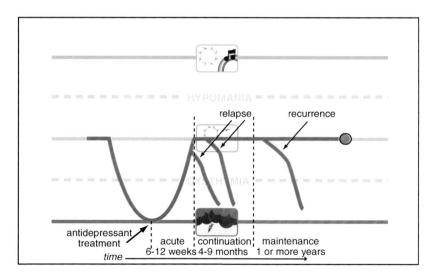

Figure 7-3. Relapse and recurrence. When depression returns before there is a full remission of symptoms or within the first several months following remission of symptoms, it is called a relapse. When depression returns after a patient has recovered, it is called a recurrence.

the pharmaceutical industry to increasingly abandon the development of new antidepressants. Even patients seem to be affected by this debate, perhaps losing their confidence in the efficacy of antidepressants, since up to a third of patients in a real clinical practice setting never fill their first antidepressant prescription, and for those who do, perhaps less than half get a second month of treatment and maybe less than a quarter get an adequate trial of 3 months or longer. One thing is for sure about antidepressants, and that is that they don't work if you don't take them. Thus, the clinical effectiveness of antidepressants in clinical practice

settings is reduced by this failure of "persistency" of treatment for a long enough period of time to give the drug a chance to work.

Whatever the cause of this controversy over the efficacy of antidepressants in clinical trials, one only needs to spend a short time in a clinical practice setting to be convinced that antidepressants are powerful therapeutic agents in many patients. Nevertheless, there have been some useful consequences of the debate on the efficacy of antidepressants, such as re-energizing the integration of psychotherapies with antidepressants, searching for new non-medication

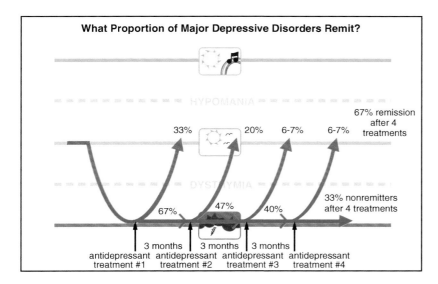

Figure 7-4. Remission rates in MDD. Approximately one-third of depressed patients will remit during treatment with any antidepressant initially. Unfortunately, for those who fail to remit, the likelihood of remission with another antidepressant monotherapy goes down with each successive trial. Thus, after a year of treatment with four sequential antidepressants taken for 12 weeks each, only two-thirds of patients will have achieved remission.

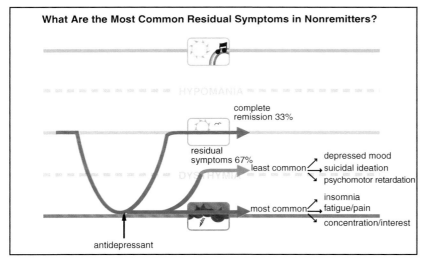

Figure 7-5. Common residual symptoms. In patients who do not achieve remission, the most common residual symptoms are insomnia, fatigue, painful physical complaints, problems concentrating, and lack of interest. The least common residual symptoms are depressed mood, suicidal ideation, and psychomotor retardation.

neurostimulation therapeutics, and studying the combination of currently available antidepressants in order to gain better outcomes, all of which will be discussed in this chapter.

How well do antidepressants work in the real world?

"Real world" trials of antidepressants tested in clinical practice settings that include patients normally excluded from marketing trials, such as the STAR*D trial of antidepressants (Sequenced Treatment Alternatives to Relieve Depression), have recently provided sobering results. Only a third of such patients remit on their first antidepressant treatment, and even after a year of treatment with a sequence of four different

antidepressants given for 12 weeks each, only about two-thirds of depressed patients achieve remission of their symptoms (Figure 7-4).

What are the most common symptoms that persist after antidepressant treatment, causing this disorder not to go into remission? The answer is shown in Figure 7-5, and the symptoms include insomnia, fatigue, multiple painful physical complaints (even though these are not part of the formal diagnostic criteria for depression), as well as problems concentrating, and lack of interest or motivation. Antidepressants appear to work fairly well in improving depressed mood, suicidal ideation, and psychomotor retardation (Figure 7-5).

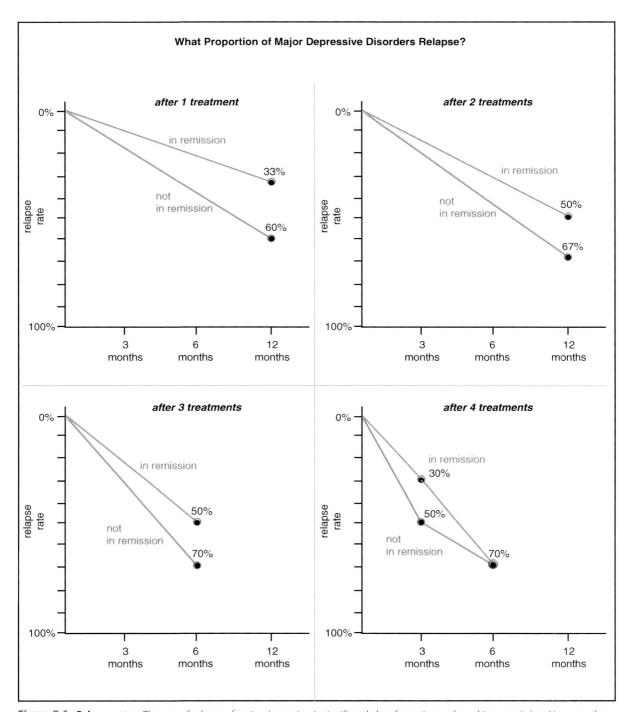

Figure 7-6. Relapse rates. The rate of relapse of major depression is significantly less for patients who achieve remission. However, there is still risk of relapse even in remitters, and the likelihood increases with the number of treatments it takes to get the patient to remit. Thus the relapse rate for patients who do not remit ranges from 60% at 12 months after one treatment to 70% at 6 months after four treatments; but for those who do remit, it ranges from only 33% at 12 months after one treatment all the way to 70% at 6 months after four treatments. In other words, the protective nature of remission virtually disappears once it takes four treatments to achieve remission.

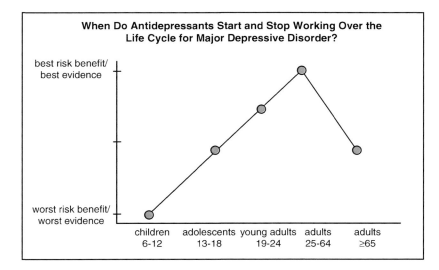

When Do Antidepressants Start and Stop Working Over the Life Cycle for Major Depressive Disorder?

best risk benefit/ best evidence

worst risk benefit/ worst evidence

| children 6-12 | adolescents 13-18 | young adults 19-24 | adults 25-64 | adults ≥65 |

Figure 7-7. Antidepressants over the life cycle. The efficacy, tolerability, and safety of antidepressants have been studied mostly in individuals between the ages of 25 and 64. Existing data across all age groups suggest that the risk–benefit ratio is most favorable for adults between the ages of 25 and 64 and somewhat less so for adults between the ages of 19 and 24, due to a possibly increased risk of suicidality in younger adults. Limited data in children and adolescents also suggest increased risk of suicidality; this, coupled with a lack of data demonstrating clear antidepressant efficacy, gives children between the ages of 6 and 12 the worst risk–benefit ratio, with adolescents intermediate between young adults and children. Elderly patients, 65 years of age and older, may not respond as well or as quickly to antidepressants as other adults and may also experience more side effects than younger adults.

Why should we care whether a patient is in remission from major depression or has just a few persistent symptoms? The answer can be found in Figure 7-6, which shows both good news and bad news about antidepressant treatment over the long run. The good news is that if an antidepressant gets your patient into remission, that patient has a significantly lower relapse rate. The bad news is that there are still very frequent relapses in the remitters, and these relapse rates get worse the more treatments the patient needs to take in order to get into remission (Figure 7-6).

Data like these have galvanized researchers and clinicians alike to treat patients to the point of remission of all symptoms whenever possible, and to try to intervene as early as possible in this illness of major depression, not only to be merciful in trying to relieve current suffering from depressive symptoms, but also because of the possibility that aggressive treatment may prevent disease progression. The concept of disease progression in major depression is controversial, unproven, and provocative, but makes a good deal of sense intuitively for many clinicians and investigators (Figure 6-23). The idea is that chronicity of major depression, development of treatment resistance, and likelihood of relapse could all be reduced, with a better overall outcome, with aggressive treatment of major depressive episodes that leads to remission of all symptoms, thus potentially modifiying the course of this illness. This may pose an especially difficult challenge for treatment of younger patients, where

risks versus benefits of antidepressants are currently debated (Figure 7-7).

Antidepressants over the life cycle

Adults between the ages of 25 and 64 might have the best chance of getting a good response and with the best tolerability to an antidepressant (Figure 7-7). Adults aged 65 or older may not respond as quickly or as robustly to antidepressants, especially if their first episode starts at this age, and especially when their presenting symptoms are lack of interest and cognitive dysfunction rather than depressed mood, but do not have increased suicidality from taking an antidepressant. At the other end of the adult age range, those younger than 25 may benefit from antidepressant efficacy but with a slightly but statistically greater risk of suicidality (but not completed suicide) (Figure 7-7). Age is thus an important consideration for whether, when, and how to treat a patient with antidepressants throughout the life cycle, and with what potential risk versus benefit.

Antidepressant classes
Blocking monoamine transporters

Classic antidepressant action is to block one or more of the transporters for serotonin, norepinephrine, and/or dopamine. This pharmacologic action is entirely consistent with the monoamine hypothesis of depression, which states that monoamines are

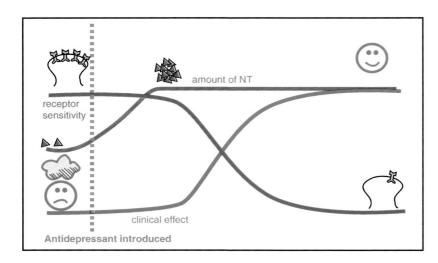

Figure 7-8. Time course of antidepressant effects. This figure depicts the different time courses for three effects of antidepressant drugs – namely, clinical changes, neurotransmitter (NT) changes, and receptor sensitivity changes. Specifically, the amount of NT changes relatively rapidly after an antidepressant is introduced. However, the clinical effect is delayed, as is the desensitization, or downregulation, of neurotransmitter receptors. This temporal correlation of clinical effects with changes in receptor sensitivity has given rise to the hypothesis that changes in neurotransmitter receptor sensitivity may actually mediate the clinical effects of antidepressant drugs. These clinical effects include not only antidepressant and anxiolytic actions but also the development of tolerance to the acute side effects of antidepressant drugs.

somehow depleted (Figure 6-34B), and when boosted with effective antidepressants relieve depression (Figure 7-8). One problem for the monoamine hypothesis, however, is that the action of antidepressants at monoamine transporters can raise monoamine levels quite rapidly in some brain areas, and certainly sooner than the antidepressant clinical effects occur in patients weeks later (Figure 7-8). How could immediate changes in neurotransmitter levels caused by antidepressants be linked to clinical actions that are much later in time? The answer may be that the acute increases in neurotransmitter levels cause adaptive changes in neurotransmitter *receptor sensitivity* in a delayed time course consistent with the onset of clinical antidepressant actions (Figure 7-8). Specifically, acutely enhanced synaptic levels of neurotransmitter (Figure 7-9A) could lead to adaptive downregulation and desensitization of postsynaptic neurotransmitter receptors over time (Figure 7-9B).

This concept of antidepressants causing changes in neurotransmitter receptor sensitivity is also consistent with the neurotransmitter receptor hypothesis of depression causing upregulation of neurotransmitter receptors in the first place (Figure 7-9A). Thus, antidepressants theoretically reverse this pathological upregulation of receptors over time (Figure 7-9B). Furthermore, the time course of receptor adaptation fits both with the onset of therapeutic effects and with the onset of tolerance to many side effects. Different receptors likely mediate these different actions, but both the onset of therapeutic action and the onset of

tolerance to side effects may occur with the same delayed time course.

Adaptive changes in receptor number or sensitivity are likely the result of alterations in gene expression (Figure 7-10). This may include not only turning off the synthesis of neurotransmitter receptors, but also increasing the synthesis of various neurotrophic factors such as BDNF (brain-derived neurotrophic factor) (Figure 7-10), as also discussed in Chapter 6 and illustrated in Figures 6-36 through 6-38. Such mechanisms may apply broadly to all effective antidepressants, and may provide a final common pathway for the action of antidepressants.

Selective serotonin reuptake inhibitors (SSRIs)

Rarely has a class of drugs transformed a field as dramatically as have the SSRIs transformed clinical psychopharmacology. Some estimate that SSRI prescriptions in the US alone occur at the rate of six prescriptions per second, 24/7, year round. Already prominent in Europe, SSRIs are now entering Japan and all across Asia, with increasing use throughout the entire world. Clinical indications for the use of SSRIs range far beyond major depressive disorder, especially to a number of anxiety disorders, and also to premenstrual dysphoric disorder, eating disorders, and beyond. There are six principal agents in this group that all share the common property of serotonin reuptake inhibition, and thus they all belong to

Neurotransmitter Receptor Hypothesis of Antidepressant Action

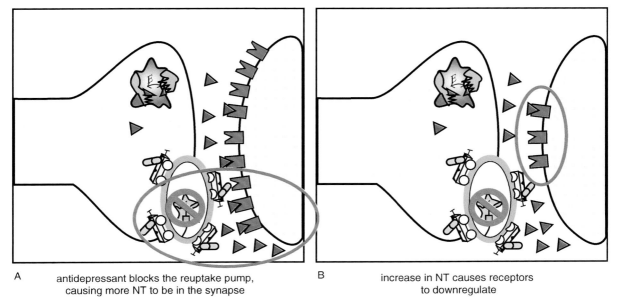

A   antidepressant blocks the reuptake pump, causing more NT to be in the synapse

B   increase in NT causes receptors to downregulate

Figure 7-9. Neurotransmitter receptor hypothesis of antidepressant action. Although antidepressants cause an immediate increase in monoamines, they do not have immediate therapeutic effects. This may be explained by the monoamine receptor hypothesis of depression, which states that depression is caused by upregulation of monoamine receptors; thus antidepressant efficacy would be related to downregulation of those receptors, as shown here. (A) When an antidepressant blocks a monoamine reuptake pump, this causes more neurotransmitter (NT) (in this case, norepinephrine) to accumulate in the synapse. (B) The increased availability of NT ultimately causes receptors to downregulate. The time course of receptor adaptation is consistent both with the delayed clinical effects of antidepressants and with development of tolerance to antidepressant side effects.

the same drug class, known as SSRIs. However, each of these six drugs also has unique pharmacological properties that allow them to be distinguished from each other. First, we will discuss what these six drugs share in common, and then we will explore their distinctive individual properties that allow sophisticated prescribers to match specific drug profiles to individual patient symptom profiles.

What the six SSRIs have in common

All six SSRIs have the same major pharmacologic feature in common: selective and potent inhibition of serotonin reuptake, also known as inhibition of the serotonin transporter or SERT (Figure 7-11). This simple concept was introduced in Chapter 5 and illustrated in Figure 5-14 and is shown here in Figure 7-12. Although the action of SSRIs at the *presynaptic axon terminal* has classically been emphasized (Figure 7-12), it now appears that events occurring at the *somatodendritic* end of the serotonin neuron (near the cell body) may be more important in explaining the therapeutic actions of the SSRIs (Figures 7-13 through 7-17). That

is, in the depressed state, the monoamine hypothesis of depression states that serotonin may be deficient, both at presynaptic somatodendritic areas near the cell body (on the left in Figure 7-13) and in the synapse itself near the axon terminal (on the right in Figure 7-13). The neurotransmitter receptor hypothesis proposes that monoamine receptors may be upregulated as shown in Figure 7-13, representing the depressed state before treatment. Neuronal firing rates may also be dysregulated in depression, contributing to regional abnormalities in information processing, and the development of specific symptoms depending upon the region affected, as discussed in Chapter 6 and shown in Figures 6-33 and 6-45.

When an SSRI is given acutely, it is well known that 5HT rises due to blockade of SERT. What is somewhat surprising, however, is that blocking the presynaptic SERT does *not* immediately lead to a great deal of serotonin in many synapses. In fact, when SSRI treatment is initiated, 5HT rises to much greater levels at the somatodendritic area located in the midbrain raphe (on the left in Figure 7-14) due to

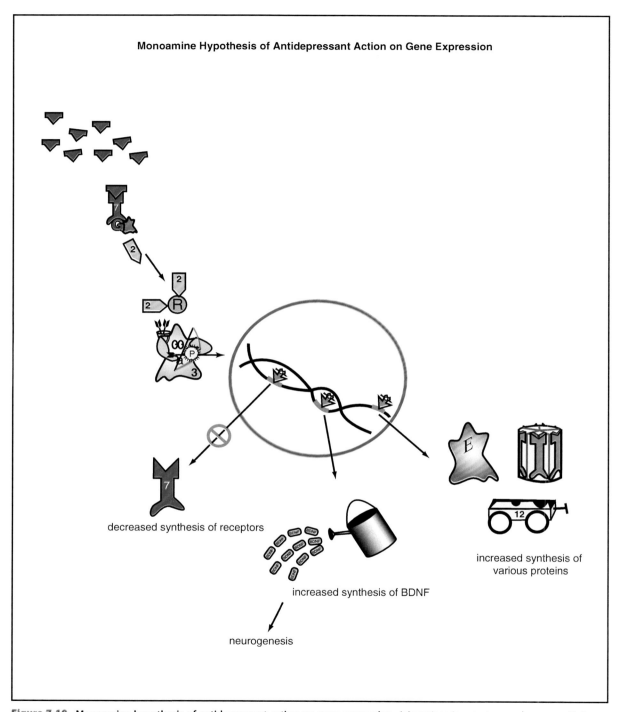

Figure 7-10. Monoamine hypothesis of antidepressant action on gene expression. Adaptations in receptor number or sensitivity are likely due to alterations in gene expression, as shown here. The neurotransmitter at the top is presumably increased by an antidepressant. The cascading consequence of this is ultimately to change the expression of critical genes in order to effect an antidepressant response. This includes downregulating some genes so that there is decreased synthesis of receptors as well as upregulating other genes so that there is increased synthesis of critical proteins, such as brain-derived neurotrophic factor (BDNF).

SSRI

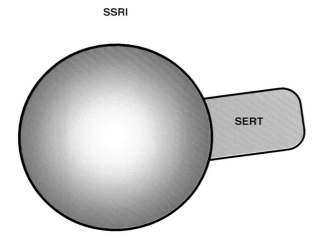

Figure 7-11. Selective serotonin reuptake inhibitors. Shown here is an icon depicting the core feature of selective serotonin reuptake inhibitors (SSRIs), namely serotonin reuptake inhibition. Although the agents in this class have unique pharmacological profiles, they all share the common property of serotonin transporter (SERT) inhibition.

SSRI Action

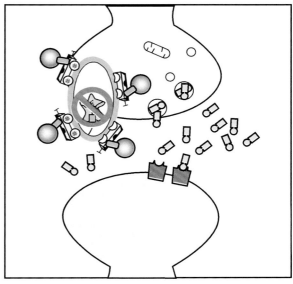

Figure 7-12. SSRI action. In this figure, the serotonin reuptake inhibitor (SRI) portion of the SSRI molecule is shown inserted into the serotonin reuptake pump (the serotonin transporter, or SERT), blocking it and causing an antidepressant effect.

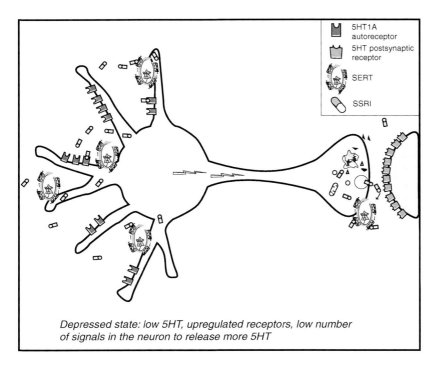

Figure 7-13. Mechanism of action of selective serotonin reuptake inhibitors (SSRIs), part 1. Depicted here is a serotonin (5HT) neuron in a depressed patient. In depression, the 5HT neuron is conceptualized as having a relative deficiency of the neurotransmitter 5HT. Also, the number of 5HT receptors is upregulated, including presynaptic 5HT$_{1A}$ autoreceptors as well as postsynaptic 5HT receptors.

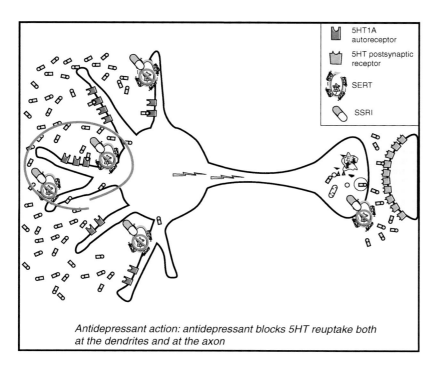

	5HT1A autoreceptor
	5HT postsynaptic receptor
	SERT
	SSRI

Figure 7-14. Mechanism of action of selective serotonin reuptake inhibitors (SSRIs), part 2. When an SSRI is administered, it immediately blocks the serotonin reuptake pump (see icon of an SSRI drug capsule blocking the reuptake pump, or serotonin transporter [SERT]). However, this causes serotonin to increase initially only in the somatodendritic area of the serotonin neuron (left) and not very much in the axon terminals (right).

Antidepressant action: antidepressant blocks 5HT reuptake both at the dendrites and at the axon

blockade of SERTs there, rather than in the areas of the brain where the axons terminate (on the right in Figure 7-14).

The somatodendritic area of the serotonin neuron is therefore where 5HT increases first (on the left in Figure 7-14). Serotonin receptors in this brain area have 5HT$_{1A}$ pharmacology as discussed in Chapter 5 and illustrated in Figure 5-25. When serotonin levels rise in the somatodendritic area, they stimulate nearby 5HT$_{1A}$ autoreceptors (also on the left in Figure 7-14). These immediate pharmacologic actions obviously cannot explain the delayed therapeutic actions of the SSRIs. However, these immediate actions may explain the side effects that are caused by the SSRIs when treatment is initiated.

Over time, the increased 5HT acting at the somatodendritic 5HT$_{1A}$ autoreceptors causes them to downregulate and become desensitized (on the left in Figure 7-15). This desensitization occurs because the increase in serotonin is recognized by these presynaptic 5HT$_{1A}$ receptors, and this information is sent to the cell nucleus of the serotonin neuron. The genome's reaction to this information is to issue instructions that cause these same receptors to become desensitized over time. The time course of

this desensitization correlates with the onset of therapeutic actions of the SSRIs.

Once the 5HT$_{1A}$ somatodendritic autoreceptors are desensitized, 5HT can no longer effectively turn off its own release. Since 5HT is no longer inhibiting its own release, the serotonin neuron is therefore disinhibited (Figure 7-16). This results in a flurry of 5HT release from axons and an increase in neuronal impulse flow (shown as lightning in Figure 7-16 and release of serotonin from the axon terminal on the right). This is just another way of saying the serotonin release is "turned on" at the axon terminals. The serotonin that now pours out of the various projections of serotonin pathways in the brain is what theoretically mediates the various therapeutic actions of the SSRIs.

While the presynaptic somatodendritic 5HT$_{1A}$ autoreceptors are desensitizing (Figure 7-15), serotonin is building up in synapses (Figure 7-16), and causes the postsynaptic serotonin receptors to desensitize as well (on the right in Figure 7-17). These various postsynaptic serotonin receptors in turn send information to the cell nucleus of the *postsynaptic* neuron that serotonin is targeting (on the far right of Figure 7-17). The reaction of the genome in the

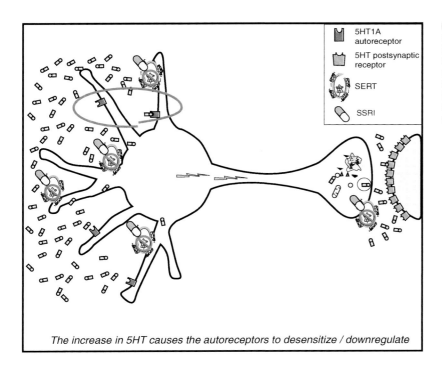

Figure 7-15. Mechanism of action of selective serotonin reuptake inhibitors (SSRIs), part 3. The consequence of serotonin increasing in the somatodendritic area of the serotonin (5HT) neuron, as depicted in Figure 7-14, is that the somatodendritic $5HT_{1A}$ autoreceptors desensitize or downregulate (red circle).

The increase in 5HT causes the autoreceptors to desensitize / downregulate

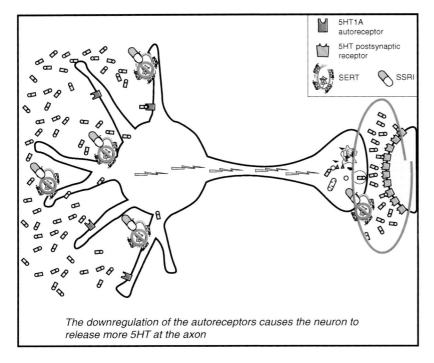

Figure 7-16. Mechanism of action of selective serotonin reuptake inhibitors (SSRIs), part 4. Once the somatodendritic receptors downregulate, as depicted in Figure 7-15, there is no longer inhibition of impulse flow in the serotonin (5HT) neuron. Thus, neuronal impulse flow is turned on. The consequence of this is release of 5HT in the axon terminal (red circle). However, this increase is delayed as compared with the increase of 5HT in the somatodendritic areas of the 5HT neuron, depicted in Figure 7-14. This delay is the result of the time it takes for somatodendritic 5HT to downregulate the $5HT_{1A}$ autoreceptors and turn on neuronal impulse flow in the 5HT neuron. This delay may explain why antidepressants do not relieve depression immediately. It is also the reason why the mechanism of action of antidepressants may be linked to increasing neuronal impulse flow in 5HT neurons, with 5HT levels increasing at axon terminals before an SSRI can exert its antidepressant effects.

The downregulation of the autoreceptors causes the neuron to release more 5HT at the axon

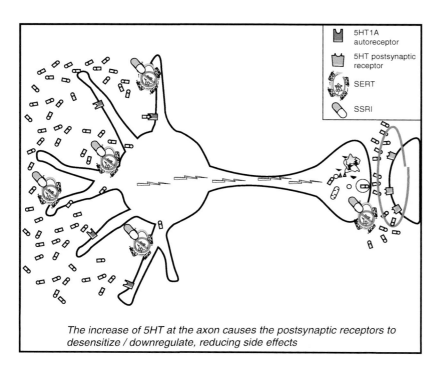

5HT1A
autoreceptor

5HT postsynaptic
receptor

SERT

SSRI

*The increase of 5HT at the axon causes the postsynaptic receptors to
desensitize / downregulate, reducing side effects*

Figure 7-17. Mechanism of action of selective serotonin reuptake inhibitors (SSRIs), part 5. Finally, once the SSRIs have blocked the reuptake pump (or serotonin transporter [SERT] in Figure 7-14), increased somatodendritic serotonin (5HT) (Figure 7-14), desensitized somatodendritic 5HT$_{1A}$ autoreceptors (Figure 7-15), turned on neuronal impulse flow (Figure 7-16), and increased release of 5HT from axon terminals (Figure 7-16), the final step (shown here) may be the desensitization of postsynaptic 5HT receptors. This desensitization may mediate the reduction of side effects of SSRIs as tolerance develops.

postsynaptic neuron is also to issue instructions to downregulate or desensitize these receptors as well. The time course of this desensitization correlates with the onset of tolerance to the side effects of the SSRIs (Figure 7-17).

This theory thus suggests a pharmacological cascading mechanism whereby the SSRIs exert their therapeutic actions: namely, powerful but delayed disinhibition of serotonin release in key pathways throughout the brain. Furthermore, side effects are hypothetically caused by the acute actions of serotonin at undesirable receptors in undesirable pathways. Finally, side effects may attenuate over time by desensitization of the very receptors that mediate them.

Unique properties of each SSRI: the not-so-selective serotonin reuptake inhibitors

Although the six SSRIs clearly share the same mechanism of action, individual patients often react very differently to one SSRI versus another. This is not generally observed in large clinical trials, where mean group differences between two SSRIs either in efficacy or in side effects are very difficult to document. Rather, such differences are seen by prescribers treating patients one at a time, with some patients experiencing a therapeutic response to one SSRI and not another, and other patients tolerating one SSRI and not another.

If blockade of SERT explains the shared clinical and pharmacological actions of SSRIs, what explains their differences? Although there is no generally accepted explanation that accounts for the commonly observed clinical phenomena of different efficacy and tolerability of various SSRIs in individual patients, it makes sense to consider those pharmacologic characteristics of the six SSRIs that are not shared with each other as candidates to explain the broad range of individual patient reactions to different SSRIs (Figures 7-18 through 7-23). Each SSRI has secondary pharmacologic actions other than SERT blockade, and no two SSRIs have identical secondary pharmacological characteristics. Whether these secondary binding profiles can account for the differences in efficacy and tolerability in individual patients remains to be proven. However, it does lead to provocative hypothesis generation and gives a rational basis for psychopharmacologists trying more than one of these agents rather than thinking "they are all the same." Sometimes only an empiric trial of different SSRIs will lead to the best match of drug to an individual patient.

Fluoxetine: an SSRI with 5HT$_{2C}$ antagonist properties

This SSRI also has 5HT$_{2C}$ antagonist actions that may explain many of its unique clinical properties (Figure 7-18). 5HT$_{2C}$ antagonism is explained in Chapter 5 and illustrated in Figures 5-52A and 5-52B. Other antidepressants with 5HT$_{2C}$ antagonist properties include mirtazapine and agomelatine; several atypical antipsychotics including quetiapine with proven antidepressant properties, as well as olanzapine, asenapine, and clozapine, also have potent 5HT$_{2C}$ antagonist actions. Blocking serotonin action at 5HT$_{2C}$ receptors disinhibits (i.e., enhances) release of both NE and DA (Figure 5-52B). 5HT$_{2C}$ antagonism may contribute not only to fluoxetine's therapeutic actions but also to its tolerability profile.

The good news about 5HT$_{2C}$ antagonism may be that it is generally activating, and many patients, even from the first dose, detect an energizing and fatigue-reducing effect of fluoxetine, with improvement in concentration and attention as well. This mechanism is perhaps best matched to depressed patients with reduced positive affect, hypersomnia, psychomotor retardation, apathy, and fatigue (Figure 6-46). Fluoxetine is also approved in some countries in combination with olanzapine for treatment-resistant unipolar depression and for bipolar depression. Since olanzapine

fluoxetine

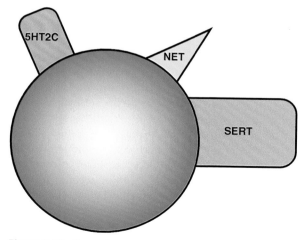

Figure 7-18. Fluoxetine. In addition to serotonin reuptake inhibition, fluoxetine has norepinephrine reuptake inhibition (NRI) and serotonin 2C (5HT$_{2C}$) antagonist actions. Fluoxetine's activating effects may be due to its actions at 5HT$_{2C}$ receptors. Norepinephrine reuptake inhibition may be clinically relevant only at very high doses. Fluoxetine is also an inhibitor at CYP 2D6 and 3A4.

also has 5HT$_{2C}$ antagonist actions (Figure 5-46), it may be that adding together the 5HT$_{2C}$ antagonist actions of both drugs could theoretically lead to further enhanced DA and NE release in cortex to mediate the antidepressant actions of this combination. 5HT$_{2C}$ antagonism may also contribute to the anti-bulimia effect of higher doses of fluoxetine, the only SSRI approved for the treatment of this eating disorder.

The bad news about 5HT$_{2C}$ antagonism is that it can be activating, so the 5HT$_{2C}$ antagonist actions of fluoxetine may contribute to this agent being sometimes less well matched to patients with agitation, insomnia, and anxiety, who may experience unwanted activation and even a panic attack if given an agent that further activates them.

Other unique properties of fluoxetine (Figure 7-18) are weak NE reuptake blocking properties that may become clinically relevant at very high doses. Fluoxetine has a long half-life (2–3 days), and its active metabolite an even longer half-life (2 weeks). The long half-life is advantageous in that it seems to reduce the withdrawal reactions that are characteristic of sudden discontinuation of some SSRIs, but it also means that it takes a long time to clear the drug and its active metabolite after discontinuing fluoxetine, and prior to starting another agent such as a monoamine oxidase inhibitor (MAOI). Fluoxetine is available not only as a once-daily formulation, but also as a once-weekly oral dosage formulation.

Sertraline: an SSRI with dopamine transporter (DAT) inhibition and σ$_1$ binding

This SSRI has two candidate mechanisms that distinguish it: dopamine transporter (DAT) inhibition and sigma-1 (σ$_1$) receptor binding (Figure 7-19). The DAT inhibitory actions are controversial since they are weaker than the SERT inhibitory actions, thus leading some experts to suggest that there is not sufficient DAT occupancy by sertraline to be clinically relevant. However, as will be discussed later in the section on norepinephrine–dopamine reuptake inhibitors (NDRIs), it is not clear that high degrees of DAT occupancy are necessary or even desirable in order to contribute to antidepressant actions. That is, perhaps only a small amount of DAT inhibition is sufficient to cause improvement in energy, motivation, and concentration, especially when added to another action such as SERT inhibition. In fact,

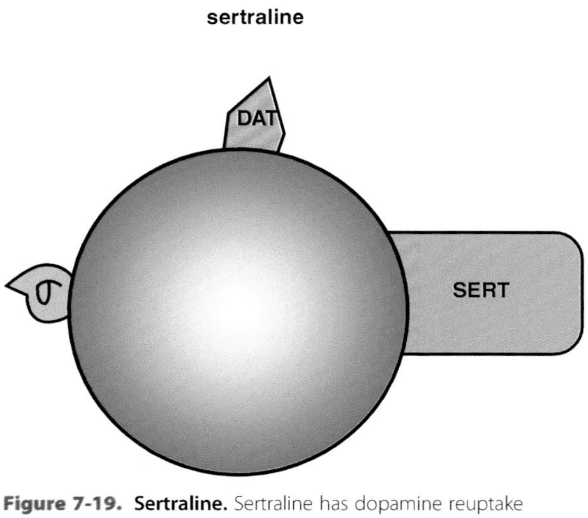

sertraline

paroxetine

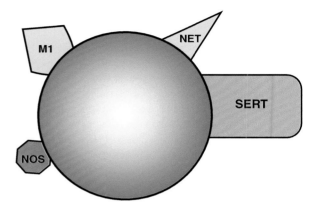

Figure 7-19. Sertraline. Sertraline has dopamine reuptake inhibition (DRI) and σ₁ receptor binding in addition to serotonin reuptake inhibition (SRI). The clinical relevance of sertraline's DRI is unknown, although it may improve energy, motivation, and concentration. Its σ properties may contribute to anxiolytic actions and may also be helpful in patients with psychotic depression.

Figure 7-20. Paroxetine. In addition to serotonin reuptake inhibition (SRI), paroxetine has mild anticholinergic actions (M₁), which can be calming or possibly sedating, weak norepinephrine reuptake inhibition (NRI), which may contribute to further antidepressant actions, and inhibition of the enzyme nitric oxide synthetase (NOS), which may contribute to sexual dysfunction. Paroxetine is also a potent inhibitor of CYP 2D6.

high-impact DAT inhibition is the property of reinforcing stimulants, including cocaine and methylphenidate, and would not generally be desired in an antidepressant.

Anecdotally, clinicians have observed the mild and desirable activating actions of sertraline in some patients with "atypical depression," improving symptoms of hypersomnia, low energy, and mood reactivity. A favorite combination of some clinicians for depressed patients is to add bupropion to sertraline (i.e., Wellbutrin to Zoloft, sometimes called "Welloft"), adding together the weak DAT inhibitory properties of each agent. Clinicians have also observed the over-activation of some patients with panic disorder by sertraline, thus requiring slower dose titration in some patients with anxiety symptoms. All of these actions of sertraline are consistent with weak DAT inhibitory actions of sertraline contributing to its clinical portfolio of actions.

The σ₁ actions of sertraline are not well understood, but might contribute to its anxiolytic effects and especially to its effects in psychotic and delusional depression, where sertraline may have advantageous therapeutic effects compared to some other SSRIs. These σ₁ actions could theoretically contribute both to anxiolytic actions and to antipsychotic actions, as will be discussed further in the section on fluvoxamine below.

Paroxetine: an SSRI with muscarinic anticholinergic and norepinephrine transporter (NET) inhibitory actions

This SSRI is preferred by many clinicians for patients with anxiety symptoms. It tends to be more calming, even sedating, early in treatment compared to the more activating actions of both fluoxetine and sertraline discussed above. Perhaps the mild anticholinergic actions of paroxetine contribute to this clinical profile (Figure 7-20). Paroxetine also has weak NET (norepinephrine transporter) inhibitory properties, which could contribute to its efficacy in depression, especially at high doses. The advantages of dual serotonin plus norepinephrine reuptake inhibiting properties, or SNRI actions, are discussed below in the section on SNRIs. It is possible that weak to moderate NET inhibition of paroxetine may contribute importantly to its antidepressant actions.

Paroxetine inhibits the enzyme nitric oxide synthetase, which could theoretically contribute to sexual dysfunction especially in men. Paroxetine is also notorious for causing withdrawal reactions upon sudden discontinuation with symptoms such as akathisia, restlessness, gastrointestinal symptoms, dizziness, and tingling, especially when suddenly discontinued from long-term high-dose treatment. This is possibly due not only to

fluvoxamine

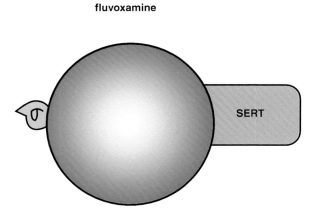

Figure 7-21. Fluvoxamine. Fluvoxamine's secondary properties include actions at σ₁ receptors, which may be anxiolytic as well as beneficial for psychotic depression, and inhibition of CYP 1A2 and 3A4.

citalopram

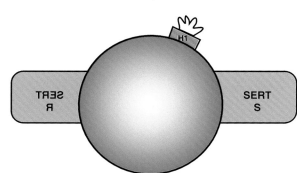

Figure 7-22. Citalopram. Citalopram consists of two enantiomers, R and S. The R enantiomer has weak antihistamine properties and is a weak inhibitor of CYP 2D6.

SERT inhibition properties, since all SSRIs can cause discontinuation reactions, but also to additional contributions from anticholinergic rebound when paroxetine is rapidly discontinued. Paroxetine is available in a controlled-release formulation, which may mitigate some of its side effects, including discontinuation reactions.

Fluvoxamine: an SSRI with σ₁ receptor binding properties

This SSRI was among the first to be launched for the treatment of depression worldwide, but was never officially approved for depression in the US, so has been considered more of an agent for the treatment of obsessive–compulsive disorder and anxiety in the US. A unique binding property of fluvoxamine, like sertraline, is its interaction at σ₁ sites, but this action is more potent for fluvoxamine than for sertraline (Figure 7-21). The physiological function of σ₁ sites is still a mystery, and thus sometimes called the "sigma enigma," but has been linked to both anxiety and psychosis. Although it is not entirely clear how to define an agonist or antagonist at σ₁ sites, recent studies suggest that fluvoxamine may be an agonist at σ₁ receptors, and that this property may contribute an additional pharmacologic action to help explain fluvoxamine's well-known anxiolytic properties. Fluvoxamine also has shown therapeutic activity in both psychotic and delusional depression, where it, like sertraline, may have advantages over other SSRIs.

Fluvoxamine is now available as a controlled-release formulation which makes once-a-day administration possible, unlike immediate-release fluvoxamine, whose shorter half-life often requires twice-daily administration. In addition, recent trials of controlled-release fluvoxamine show impressive remission rates in both obsessive–compulsive disorder and social anxiety disorder, as well as possibly less peak dose sedation.

Citalopram: an SSRI with a "good" and a "bad" enantiomer

This SSRI is comprised of two enantiomers, R and S, one of which is the mirror image of the other (Figure 7-22). The mixture of these enantiomers is known as racemic citalopram, or commonly just as citalopram, and it has mild antihistaminic properties that reside in the R enantiomer (Figure 7-22). Racemic citalopram is generally one of the better-tolerated SSRIs, and has favorable findings in the treatment of depression in the elderly, but has a somewhat inconsistent therapeutic action at the lowest dose, often requiring dose increase to optimize treatment. However, dose increase is limited due to the potential for QTc prolongation. These findings all suggest that it is not favorable for citalopram to contain the R enantiomer. In fact, some pharmacologic evidence suggests that the R enantiomer may be pharmacologically active at SERT in a manner that does not inhibit SERT but actually interferes with the ability of the active S enantiomer to inhibit SERT. This could lead to reduced inhibition of SERT, reduced synaptic 5HT, and possibly reduced net therapeutic actions, especially at low doses.

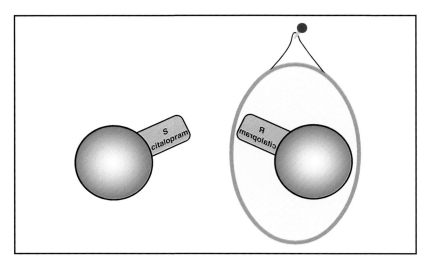

Figure 7-23. Escitalopram. The R and S enantiomers of citalopram are mirror images of each other but have slightly different clinical properties. The R enantiomer is the one with weak antihistamine properties and weak inhibition of CYP 2D6, while the S enantiomer does not have these properties. The R and S enantiomers may also differ in their effects at the serotonin transporter. The S enantiomer of citalopram has been developed and marketed as the antidepressant escitalopram.

Escitalopram: the quintessential SSRI

The solution to improving the properties of racemic citalopram is to remove the unwanted R enantiomer. The resulting drug is known as escitalopram, as it is composed of only the pure active S enantiomer (Figure 7-23). This maneuver appears to remove the antihistaminic properties, and there are no higher dose restrictions to avoid QTc prolongation. In addition, removal of the potentially interfering R isomer makes the lowest dose of escitalopram more predictably efficacious. Escitalopram is therefore the SSRI for which pure SERT inhibition is most likely to explain almost all of its pharmacologic actions. Escitalopram is considered perhaps the best-tolerated SSRI, with the fewest CYP-mediated drug interactions.

Serotonin partial agonist/reuptake inhibitors (SPARIs)

A new antidepressant introduced in the US is vilazodone, which combines SERT inhibition with a second property: $5HT_{1A}$ partial agonism. For this reason, vilazodone is called a SPARI (serotonin partial agonist/reuptake inhibitor) (Figure 7-24). The combination of serotonin reuptake inhibition with $5HT_{1A}$ partial agonism has long been known by clinicians to enhance the antidepressant properties and tolerability of SSRIs/SNRIs in some patients. Although vilazodone is the only approved agent selective for just these two actions, SERT inhibition combined

vilazodone

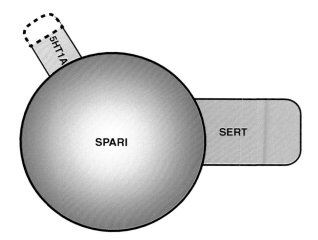

serotonin partial agonist/reuptake inhibitor

Figure 7-24. Vilazodone. Vilazodone is a partial agonist at the $5HT_{1A}$ receptor and also inhibits serotonin reuptake; thus, it is referred to as a serotonin partial agonist/reuptake inhibitor (SPARI). Its effects at $5HT_{1A}$ receptors are equal to or more potent than its effects at serotonin transporters.

with $5HT_{1A}$ partial agonism has been achieved in the past by adding atypical antipsychotics with $5HT_{1A}$ partial agonist actions such as quetiapine or aripiprazole to SSRIs/SNRIs (discussed in Chapter 5: see Figures 5-47 and 5-62). Vilazodone administration, however, is not completely identical to this option since atypical antipsychotics have many additional pharmacologic actions, some desirable and others not (Figures 5-47 and 5-62).

$5HT_{1A}$ partial agonist actions plus SERT inhibition can also be attained by augmenting SSRIs/SNRIs with the $5HT_{1A}$ partial agonist buspirone. However, this is not identical to the actions of vilazodone since buspirone and its active metabolite 6-hydroxybuspirone are weaker $5HT_{1A}$ partial agonists than vilazodone and are estimated to occupy fewer $5HT_{1A}$ receptors for a shorter time at clinically administered doses than does vilazodone. Buspirone and 6-hydroxybuspirone also bind to $5HT_{1A}$ receptors with lower affinity than $5HT$ itself, whereas vilazodone binds to $5HT_{1A}$ receptors with higher affinity than $5HT$. This suggests that administration of buspirone as an augmenting agent to an SSRI/SNRI likely results in $5HT_{1A}$ receptor occupancy that occurs more robustly in states of low $5HT$ levels and not as robustly in states of high $5HT$ levels, whereas administration of vilazodone results in binding to $5HT_{1A}$ receptors even in the presence of $5HT$. Another difference between buspirone plus an SSRI/SNRI versus vilazodone is that when buspirone augments an SSRI, the buspirone is generally dosed so that about 10–20% of $5HT_{1A}$ receptors are occupied

and the SSRI is dosed so that about 80% of SERTs are blocked. On the other hand, human neuroimaging studies suggest that vilazodone is dosed so that about 50% of both SERTs and $5HT_{1A}$ receptors are occupied. Whether this accounts for clinically significant differences between the administration of vilazodone monotherapy and the augmentation of SSRIs/SNRIs with buspirone is not known, but it could account for the apparent lesser incidence of sexual dysfunction with vilazodone than with either SSRIs alone or with the augmentation of SSRIs with buspirone. It is not known whether the enhanced efficacy of buspirone combined with SSRIs for depression demonstrated in clinical trials for patients who fail SSRI monotherapy also applies to vilazodone, as appropriate clinical trials to determine this have not yet been conducted. In animal models, adding $5HT_{1A}$ partial agonism to SSRIs causes more immediate and robust elevations of brain $5HT$ levels than SSRIs do alone. This is thought to be due to the fact that $5HT_{1A}$ partial agonists are a type of "artificial serotonin" selective especially for presynaptic somatodendritic $5HT_{1A}$ autoreceptors, and that $5HT_{1A}$ partial agonist action occurs immediately after drug is given (Figure 7-25). Thus, $5HT_{1A}$ immediate partial agonist actions are theoretically additive or

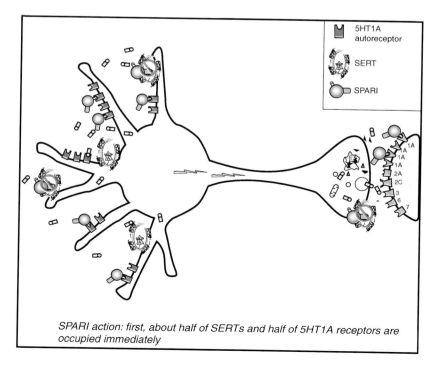

5HT1A
autoreceptor

SERT

SPARI

Figure 7-25. Mechanism of action of serotonin partial agonist/reuptake inhibitors (SPARIs), part 1. When a SPARI is administered, about half of serotonin transporters (SERTs) and half of serotonin 1A ($5HT_{1A}$) receptors are occupied immediately.

SPARI action: first, about half of SERTs and half of 5HT1A receptors are occupied immediately

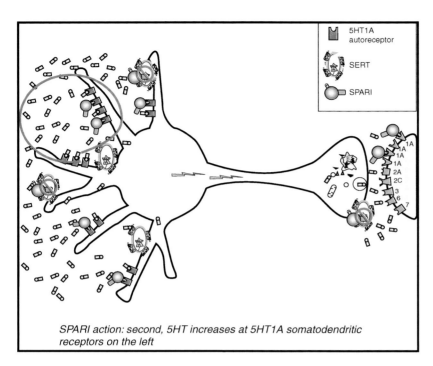

Figure 7-26. Mechanism of action of serotonin partial agonist/reuptake inhibitors (SPARIs), part 2. Blockade of the serotonin transporter (SERT) causes serotonin to increase initially in the somatodendritic area of the serotonin neuron (left).

SPARI action: second, 5HT increases at 5HT1A somatodendritic receptors on the left

synergistic with simultaneous SERT inhibition, since this leads to faster and more robust actions at $5HT_{1A}$ somatodendritic autoreceptors (Figure 7-26) than with SERT inhibition alone (Figure 7-14), including their downregulation (Figure 7-27). This hypothetically causes faster and more robust elevation of synaptic 5HT (Figure 7-28) than is possible with SSRIs alone (Figure 7-16). In addition, $5HT_{1A}$ partial agonism with vilazodone's SPARI mechanism occurs immediately at postsynaptic $5HT_{1A}$ receptors (Figure 7-26), with actions at these receptors that are thus faster and with a different type of stimulation compared to the delayed full agonist actions of serotonin itself when increased by SERT inhibition alone (Figure 7-16). The downstream actions of $5HT_{1A}$ receptors that lead to enhanced dopamine release (Figure 7-29), discussed in Chapter 5 and illustrated in Figures 5-15C and 5-16C, may be hypothetically responsible for the observed reduction in sexual dysfunction seen in patients with the combination of SERT inhibition plus $5HT_{1A}$ partial agonist actions compared to SERT inhibition alone.

Theoretically, SPARI actions could lead to faster antidepressant onset, if rapid elevation of 5HT is linked to rapid antidepressant onset. However,

clinical studies do not support this, because the rapid increase in serotonin is not well tolerated, due especially to gastrointestinal side effects, and dose titration must be slowed down in order to attain full dosing, also slowing down any potential rapid antidepressant onset. SPARI actions could hypothetically lead to more antidepressant efficacy than selective SERT inhibition, as suggested by buspirone augmentation of SSRIs, but this has not been demonstrated yet in head-to-head trials of vilazodone against an SSRI. Finally, SPARI actions could theoretically lead to less sexual dysfunction, due to lesser degrees of SERT inhibition than SSRIs plus favorable downstream dopaminergic actions. Low sexual dysfunction is shown for vilazodone in placebo-controlled trials but not yet proven to be less than that associated with SSRIs in head-to-head trials.

Serotonin–norepinephrine reuptake inhibitors (SNRIs)

SNRIs combine the robust SERT inhibition of the SSRIs with various degrees of inhibition of the norepinephrine transporter (or NET) (Figures 7-30

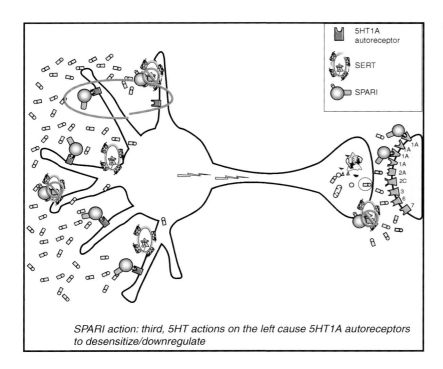

SPARI action: third, 5HT actions on the left cause 5HT1A autoreceptors to desensitize/downregulate

Figure 7-27. **Mechanism of action of serotonin partial agonist/reuptake inhibitors (SPARIs), part 3.** The consequence of serotonin increasing in the somatodendritic area of the serotonin (5HT) neuron, as depicted in Figure 7-26, is that the somatodendritic 5HT$_{1A}$ autoreceptors desensitize or downregulate (red circle).

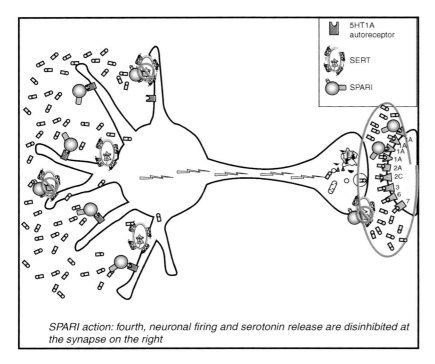

SPARI action: fourth, neuronal firing and serotonin release are disinhibited at the synapse on the right

Figure 7-28. **Mechanism of action of serotonin partial agonist/reuptake inhibitors (SPARIs), part 4.** Once the somatodendritic receptors downregulate, as depicted in Figure 7-27, there is no longer inhibition of impulse flow in the serotonin (5HT) neuron. Thus, neuronal impulse flow is turned on. The consequence of this is release of 5HT in the axon terminal (red circle).

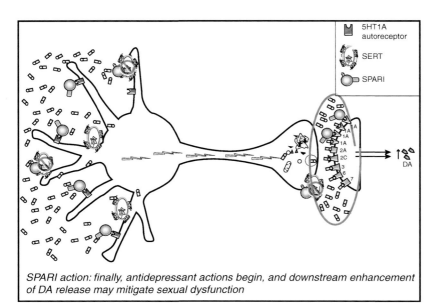

Figure 7-29. Mechanism of action of serotonin partial agonist/reuptake inhibitors (SPARIs), part 5. Finally, once the SPARIs have blocked the serotonin transporter (SERT) (Figure 7-25], increased somatodendritic serotonin (5HT) (Figure 7-26), desensitized somatodendritic 5HT$_{1A}$ autoreceptors (Figure 7-27), turned on neuronal impulse flow (Figure 7-28), and increased release of 5HT from axon terminals (Figure 7-28), the final step (shown here, red circle) may be the desensitization of postsynaptic 5HT receptors. This timeframe correlates with antidepressant action. In addition, the predominance of 5HT$_{1A}$ actions may lead to downstream enhancement of dopamine (DA) release, which may mitigate sexual dysfunction.

SPARI action: finally, antidepressant actions begin, and downstream enhancement of DA release may mitigate sexual dysfunction

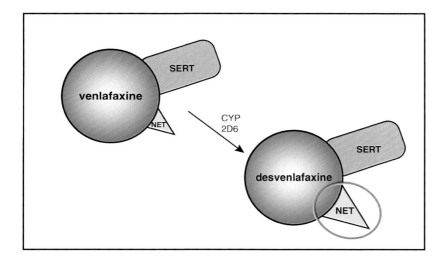

Figure 7-30. **Venlafaxine and desvenlafaxine.** Venlafaxine inhibits reuptake of both serotonin (SRI) and norepinephrine (NRI), thus combining two therapeutic mechanisms in one agent. Venlafaxine's serotonergic actions are present at low doses, while its noradrenergic actions are progressively enhanced as dose increases. Venlafaxine is converted to its active metabolite, desvenlafaxine, by CYP 2D6. Like venlafaxine, desvenlafaxine inhibits reuptake of serotonin (SRI) and norepinephrine (NRI), but its NRI actions are greater relative to its SRI actions compared to venlafaxine. Venlafaxine administration usually results in plasma levels of venlafaxine that are about half those of desvenlafaxine; however, this can vary depending on genetic polymorphisms of CYP 2D6 and whether patients are taking drugs that are inhibitors or inducers of CYP 2D6. Thus the degree of NET inhibition with venlafaxine administration may be unpredictable. Desvenlafaxine has now been developed as a separate drug. It has relatively greater norepinephrine reuptake inhibition (NRI) than venlafaxine but is still more potent at the serotonin transporter.

through 7-33). Theoretically, there should be some therapeutic advantage of adding NET inhibition to SERT inhibition, since one mechanism may add efficacy to the other mechanism by widening the reach of these antidepressants to the monoamine neurotransmitter systems throughout more brain regions. A practical indication that dual monoamine mechanisms may lead to more efficacy is the finding that the SNRI venlafaxine frequently seems to have greater antidepressant efficacy as the dose increases,

duloxetine

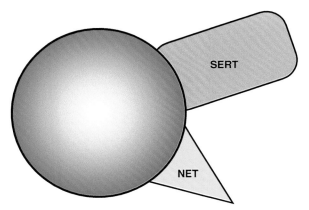

Figure 7-31. Duloxetine. Duloxetine inhibits reuptake of both serotonin (SRI) and norepinephrine (NRI). Its noradrenergic actions may contribute to efficacy for painful physical symptoms. Duloxetine is also an inhibitor of CYP 2D6.

milnacipran

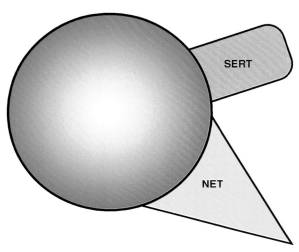

Figure 7-32. Milnacipran. Milnacipran inhibits reuptake of both serotonin (SRI) and norepinephrine (NRI) but is a more potent inhibitor of the norepinephrine transporter (NET) than the serotonin transporter (SERT). Its robust NET inhibition may contribute to efficacy for painful physical symptoms.

theoretically due to recruiting more and more NET inhibition as the dose is raised (i.e., the noradrenergic "boost"). Clinicians and experts currently debate whether remission rates are higher with SNRIs compared to SSRIs or whether SNRIs are more helpful than other options in depressed patients who fail to respond to SSRIs. One area where SNRIs have established clear efficacy but SSRIs have not is in the treatment of multiple pain syndromes. SNRIs also may have greater efficacy than SSRIs in the treatment of vasomotor symptoms associated with perimenopause, although this is not as well established.

NET inhibition increases DA in prefrontal cortex

Although SNRIs are commonly called "dual action" serotonin–norepinephrine agents, they actually have a third action on dopamine in the prefrontal cortex, but not elsewhere in the brain. Thus, they are not "full" triple action agents since they do not inhibit the dopamine transporter (DAT), but SNRIs can perhaps be considered to have "two-and-a-half" actions, rather than just two. That is, SNRIs not only boost serotonin and norepinephrine throughout the brain (Figure 7-33), but they also boost dopamine specifically in prefrontal cortex (Figure 7-34). This third mechanism of boosting dopamine in an important area of the brain associated with several symptoms of depression should add another theoretical advantage to the pharmacology of SNRIs and to their efficacy in the treatment of major depression.

How does NET inhibition boost DA in prefrontal cortex? The answer is illustrated in Figure 7-34. In prefrontal cortex, SERTs and NETs are present in abundance on serotonin and norepinephrine nerve terminals, respectively, but there are very few DATs on dopamine nerve terminals in this part of the brain (Figure 7-34). The consequence of this is that once DA is released, it is free to cruise away from the synapse (Figure 7-34A). The diffusion radius of DA is thus wider (Figure 7-34A) than is the diffusion radius of NE in prefrontal cortex (Figure 7-34B), since there is NET at the NE synapse (Figure 7-34B) but no DAT at the DA synapse (Figure 7-34A). This arrangement may enhance the regulatory importance of dopamine in prefrontal cortex functioning, since DA in this part of the brain can interact with DA receptors not only at its own synapse but at a distance, perhaps enhancing the ability of DA to regulate cognition in an entire area within its diffusion radius, not just at a single synapse. This was discussed in Chapter 1 and illustrated in Figure 1-7.

Dopamine action is therefore not terminated by DAT in prefrontal cortex, but by two other mechanisms. That is, DA diffuses away from the DA synapse until it either encounters the enzyme COMT (catchol-*O*-methyl-transferase), which degrades it

SNRI Action

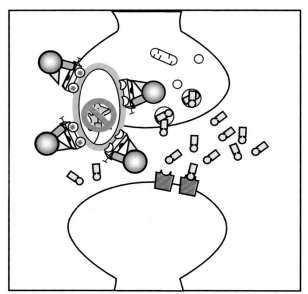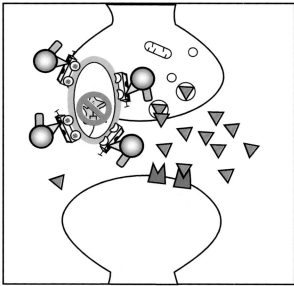

Figure 7-33. SNRI actions. In this figure, the dual actions of the serotonin–norepinephrine reuptake inhibitors (SNRIs) are shown. Both the serotonin reuptake inhibitor (SRI) portion of the SNRI molecule (left panel) and the norepinephrine reuptake inhibitor (NRI) portion of the SNRI molecule (right panel) are inserted into their respective reuptake pumps. Consequently, both pumps are blocked, and the drug mediates an antidepressant effect.

(see Figure 4-6), or until it encounters a norepinephrine reuptake pump, or NET, which transports it into the NE neuron (Figure 7-34A). NETs in fact have a greater affinity for DA than they do for NE, so they will pump DA as well as NE into NE nerve terminals, halting the action of either.

What is interesting is to see what happens when NET is inhibited in prefrontal cortex. As expected, NET inhibition enhances synaptic NE levels and increases the diffusion radius of NE (Figure 7-34B). Somewhat surprising may be that NET inhibition also enhances DA levels and increases DA's diffusion radius (Figure 7-34C). The bottom line is that NET inhibition increases both NE and DA in prefrontal cortex. Thus, SNRIs have "two-and-a-half" mechanisms: boosting serotonin throughout the brain, boosting norepinephrine throughout the brain and boosting dopamine in prefrontal cortex (but not in other DA projection areas).

Venlafaxine

Depending upon the dose, venlafaxine has different degrees of inhibition of 5HT reuptake (most potent and robust even at low doses), versus NE reuptake (moderate potency and robust only at higher doses) (Figure 7-30). However, there are no significant actions on other receptors. It remains controversial whether venlafaxine or other SNRIs have greater efficacy in major depression than SSRIs, either in terms of enhanced remission rates, more robust sustained remission over long-term treatment, or greater efficacy for treatment-resistant depression – but it seems plausible, given the two mechanisms and the boosting of two monoamines. Venlafaxine is approved and widely used for several anxiety disorders as well. Adding NET inhibition likely accounts for two side effects of venlafaxine in some patients, sweating and elevated blood pressure.

Venlafaxine is available as an extended-release formulation (venlafaxine XR), which not only allows for once-daily administration, but also significantly reduces side effects, especially nausea. In contrast to several other psychotropic drugs available in controlled-release formulations, venlafaxine XR is a considerable improvement over the immediate-release formulation. The immediate-release formulation of venlafaxine has actually fallen into little or no use because of unacceptable nausea and other side effects associated with this formulation, especially when venlafaxine immediate-release is started or when it is stopped. However, venlafaxine even in controlled-release formulation can cause

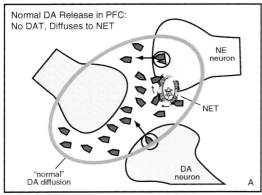

Normal DA Release in PFC:
No DAT, Diffuses to NET

NE
neuron

NET

"normal"
DA diffusion

DA
neuron

A

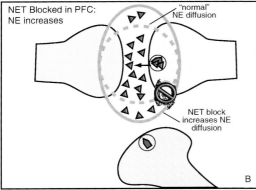

NET Blocked in PFC:
NE increases

"normal"
NE diffusion

NET block
increases NE
diffusion

B

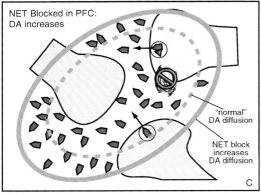

NET Blocked in PFC:
DA increases

"normal"
DA diffusion

NET block
increases
DA diffusion

C

Figure 7-34. Norepinephrine transporter blockade and dopamine in the prefrontal cortex. (A) Although there are abundant serotonin transporters (SERTs) and norepinephrine transporters (NETs) in the prefrontal cortex (PFC), there are very few dopamine transporters (DATs). This means that dopamine can diffuse away from the synapse and therefore exert its actions within a larger radius. Dopamine's actions are terminated at norepinephrine axon terminals, because DA is taken up by NET. (B) NET blockade in the prefrontal cortex leads to an increase in synaptic norepinephrine, thus increasing norepinephrine's diffusion radius. (C) Because NET takes up dopamine as well as norepinephrine, NET blockade also leads to an increase in synaptic dopamine, further increasing its diffusion radius. Thus, agents that block NET increase norepinephrine throughout the brain and both norepinephrine and dopamine in the prefrontal cortex.

withdrawal reactions, sometimes quite bothersome, especially after sudden discontinuation from high-dose long-term treatment. Nevertheless, the controlled-release formulation is highly preferred because of enhanced tolerability.

Desvenlafaxine

Venlafaxine is a substrate for CYP 2D6, which converts it to an active metabolite desvenlafaxine (Figure 7-30). Desvenlafaxine has greater NET inhibition relative to SERT inhibition compared to venlafaxine. Normally, after venlafaxine administration, the plasma levels of venlafaxine are about half of those for desvenlafaxine. However, this is highly variable, depending upon whether the patient is taking another drug that is a CYP 2D6 inhibitor, which shifts the plasma levels towards more venlafaxine and less desvenlafaxine, also reducing the relative amount of NET inhibition. Variability in plasma levels of venlafaxine versus desvenlafaxine is also due to genetic polymorphisms for CYP 2D6, such that poor metabolizers will shift the ratio of these two drugs towards more parent venlafaxine and away from the active metabolite desvenlafaxine, and thus reduce the relative amount of NET inhibition. As a result of these considerations, is can be somewhat unpredictable how much NET inhibition a given dose of venlafaxine will have in a given patient at a given time, whereas this is more predictable for desvenlafaxine. Expert clinicians have learned to solve this problem with skilled dose titration of venlafaxine, but the recent development of desvenlafaxine as a separate drug may also solve this problem with less need for dose titration and more consistent NET inhibition at a given dose across all patients.

Studies of desvenlafaxine have reported efficacy in reducing vasomotor symptoms (VMS) in perimenopausal women, whether they are depressed or not. Early studies have shown promising, if inconsistent, results for VMS with some SSRIs, as well as with the α_2 agonist clonidine and even the anticonvulsant/chronic pain agent gabapentin. However, the most promising results to date seem to be with SNRIs, especially the SNRI desvenlafaxine.

Many perimenopausal women develop hot flushes and other VMS, including night sweats, insomnia, and even depression, but do not wish to undergo estrogen replacement therapy (ERT). Desvenlafaxine appears to have efficacy in reducing VMS in such women and may provide an alternative to ERT for these women. However, it is not formally approved for this use despite several positive studies. It may be important to treat VMS not only because they are distressing in and of themselves, but also because they may be a harbinger of onset or relapse of major depression. Hypothetically, fluctuating estrogen levels not only can cause VMS, but also can be a physiological trigger for major depressive episodes during perimenopause. Dysregulation of neurotransmitter systems within hypothalamic thermoregulatory centers by irregular fluctuation of estrogen levels could lead to neurotransmitter deficiencies that trigger both VMS and depression. It is thus not surprising that other symptoms related to dysregulation of neurotransmitters within the hypothalamus can occur in both perimenopause and in depression, namely insomnia, weight gain, and decreased libido.

Postmenopausally, despite the lack of chaotic estrogen fluctuations, many women continue to experience VMS. This may be due to the loss of expression of sufficient numbers of brain glucose transporters due to low concentrations of estrogen. Theoretically, this would cause inefficient CNS transport of glucose, which would be detected in hypothalamic centers that would react by triggering a noradrenergic alarm, with vasomotor response, increase blood flow to the brain, and compensatory increase in brain glucose transport. Presumably, SNRI treatment could reduce an over-reactive hypothalamus and reduce consequent vasomotor symptoms. One issue of note relates to the observation that SSRIs seem to work better in women in the presence of estrogen than in the absence of estrogen. Thus, SSRIs may have more reliable efficacy in premenopausal women (who have normal cycling estrogen levels) and in postmenopausal women who are undergoing ERT than in postmenopausal women who are not taking ERT. By contrast, SNRIs seem to have consistent efficacy in both pre- and postmenopausal women, and in postmenopausal women whether they are undergoing ERT or not. Thus, the treatment of depression in postmenopausal women should take into consideration whether they have vasomotor symptoms, and whether they are taking ERT, before deciding whether to prescribe an SSRI or an SNRI.

Duloxetine

This SNRI, characterized pharmacologically by slightly more potent SERT than NET inhibition (Figure 7-31), has transformed how we think about depression and pain. Classic teaching was that depression caused pain that was psychic (as in "I feel your pain") and not somatic (as in "ouch"), and that psychic pain was secondary to emotional suffering in depression; therefore, it was thought, anything that made depression better would make psychic pain better nonspecifically. Somatic pain was conceptualized classically as different from psychic pain in depression, due to something wrong with the body and not due to something wrong with emotions. Somatic pain was thus not thought to be caused by depression, although depression could supposedly make it worse, and classically somatic pain was not treated with antidepressants.

Studies with duloxetine have changed all this. Not only does this SNRI relieve depression in the absence of pain, but it also relieves pain in the absence of depression. All sorts of pain are improved by duloxetine, from diabetic peripheral neuropathic pain, to fibromyalgia, to chronic musculoskeletal pain such as that associated with osteoarthritis and low back problems. These findings of the efficacy of duloxetine for multiple pain syndromes have also validated that painful physical (somatic) symptoms are a legitimate set of symptoms that accompany depression, and are not just a form of emotional pain. The use of SNRIs such as duloxetine in pain syndromes is discussed in Chapter 10. So, duloxetine has established efficacy not only in depression and in chronic pain, but also in patients with chronic painful physical symptoms of depression. Painful physical symptoms are frequently ignored or missed by patients and clinicians alike in the setting of major depression, and until recently the link of these symptoms to major depression was not well appreciated, in part because painful physical symptoms are not included in the list of symptoms for the formal diagnostic criteria for depression. Nevertheless, it is now widely appreciated that painful physical symptoms are frequently associated with a major depressive episode, and are also one of the leading residual symptoms after treatment with an antidepressant (Figure 7-5). It appears that the dual SNRI actions of duloxetine and other SNRIs are superior to the selective serotonergic actions of SSRIs for treatment of conditions such as neuropathic pain of diabetes and chronic painful physical symptoms associated with depression. The role of NET inhibition seems to be critical not only for the treatment of painful conditions without depression, but also for painful physical symptoms associated with depression. Duloxetine has also shown efficacy in the treatment of cognitive symptoms of depression that are prominent in geriatric depression, possibly exploiting the pro-noradrenergic and pro-dopaminergic consequences of NET inhibition in prefrontal cortex (Figure 7-34).

Duloxetine can be given once a day, but this is usually only a good idea after the patient has had a chance to become tolerant to it after initiating it at twice-daily dosing, especially during titration to higher doses. Duloxetine may have a lower incidence of hypertension and milder withdrawal reactions than venlafaxine.

Milnacipran

Milnacipran is the first SNRI marketed in Japan and many European countries such as France, where it is currently marketed as an antidepressant. In the US, milnacipran is not approved for depression, but is approved for fibromyalgia. Interestingly, milnacipran is not approved for the treatment of fibromyalgia in Europe. Milnacipran is a bit different from other SNRIs in that it is a relatively more potent NET than SERT inhibitor (Figure 7-32), whereas the others are more potent SERT than NET inhibitors (Figures 7-30 and 7-31). This unique pharmacologic profile may explain milnacipran's somewhat different clinical profile compared to other SNRIs. Since noradrenergic actions may be equally or more important for treatment of pain-related conditions compared to serotonergic actions, the robust NET inhibition of milnacipran suggests that it may be particularly useful in chronic pain-related conditions, not just fibromyalgia where it is approved, but possibly as well for the painful physical symptoms associated with depression and chronic neuropathic pain.

Milnacipran's potent NET inhibition also suggests a potentially favorable pharmacologic profile for the treatment of cognitive symptoms, including cognitive symptoms of depression as well as cognitive symptoms frequently associated with fibromyalgia, sometimes called "fibro-fog." Other clinical observations possibly linked to milnacipran's robust NET inhibition are that it can be more energizing and activating than other SNRIs. Common residual symptoms after treatment with an SSRI include not only cognitive symptoms, but also fatigue, lack of energy, and lack of interest, among other symptoms (Figure 7-5). An active enantiomer, levo-milnacipran, is in clinical development as an antidepressant, and is targeting fatigue and lack of energy as a potential clinical advantage due to its more potent NET inhibition.

NET inhibition may be related to observations that milnacipran may cause more sweating and urinary hesitancy than some other SNRIs. For patients with urinary hesitancy, generally due theoretically to robust pro-noradrenergic actions at bladder α_1 receptors, an α_1 antagonist can reduce these symptoms. Milnacipran must generally be given twice daily, because of its shorter half-life.

Norepinephrine–dopamine reuptake inhibitors (NDRIs): bupropion

For many years, the mechanism of action of bupropion has been somewhat unclear, and it still remains controversial among some experts. The leading hypothesis for bupropion's mechanism of action is that it inhibits the reuptake of both dopamine (i.e., dopamine transporter or DAT inhibitor) and norepinephrine (i.e., norepinephrine transporter or NET inhibitor) (Figures 7-35 and 7-36). No other specific or potent pharmacologic actions have been consistently identified for this agent.

Bupropion is metabolized to a number of active metabolites, some of which are not only more potent NET inhibitors than bupropion itself and equally potent DAT inhibitors, but are also concentrated in the brain. In some ways, therefore, bupropion is both an active

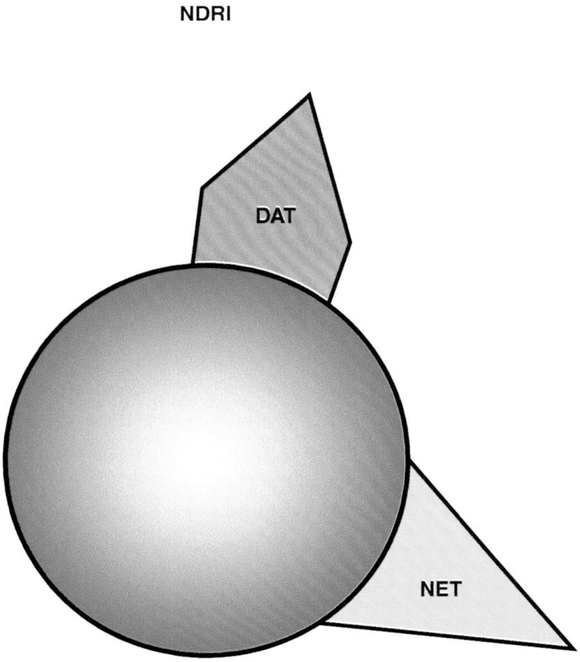

NDRI

Figure 7-35. Icon of a norepinephrine–dopamine reuptake inhibitor (NDRI). Another class of antidepressant consists of norepinephrine–dopamine reuptake inhibitors (NDRIs), for which the prototypical agent is bupropion. Bupropion has weak reuptake blocking properties for dopamine (DRI) and norepinephrine (NRI) but is an efficacious antidepressant, which may be explained in part by the more potent inhibitory properties of its metabolites.

NDRI Action

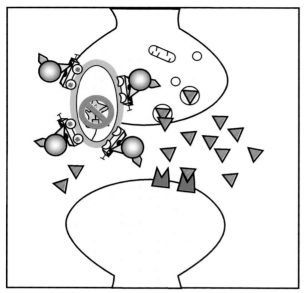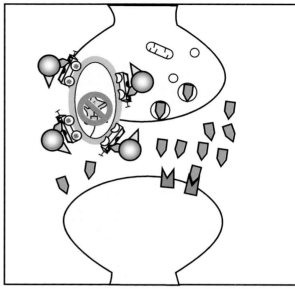

Figure 7-36. NDRI actions. In this figure the norepinephrine reuptake inhibitor (NRI) portion of the NDRI molecule (left panel) and the dopamine reuptake inhibitor (DRI) portion of the NDRI molecule (right panel) are inserted into their respective reuptake pumps. Consequently both pumps are blocked, and the drug mediates an antidepressant effect.

drug and a precursor for other active drugs (i.e., a prodrug for multiple active metabolites). The most potent of these is the + enantiomer of the 6-hydroxy metabolite of bupropion, also known as radafaxine.

Can the net effects of bupropion on NET (Figure 7-37A and B) and DAT (Figure 7-37C) account for its clinical actions in depressed patients at therapeutic doses? If one believes that 90% transporter occupancy of DAT and NET are required for antidepressant actions, the answer would be "no." Human PET scans suggest that no more than 20–30% and perhaps as little as 10–15% of striatal DATs may be occupied at therapeutic doses of bupropion. NET occupancy would be expected to be in this same range. Is this enough to explain bupropion's antidepressant actions?

Whereas it is clear from many research studies that SSRIs must be dosed to occupy a substantial fraction of SERT, perhaps up to 80 or 90% of these transporters, in order to be effective antidepressants, this is far less clear for NET or DAT occupancy, particularly in the case of drugs with an additional pharmacologic mechanism that may be synergistic with NET or DAT inhibition. That is, when most SNRIs are given in doses that occupy 80–90% of SERT, substantially fewer NETs are occupied, yet there is evidence of both additional therapeutic

actions and NE-mediated side effects of these agents with perhaps as little as 50% NET occupancy.

Furthermore, there appears to be such a thing as "too much DAT occupancy." That is, when 50% or more of DATs are occupied rapidly and briefly, this can lead to unwanted clinical actions, such as euphoria and reinforcement. In fact, rapid, short-lasting and high degrees of DAT occupancy is the pharmacologic characteristic of abusable stimulants such as cocaine and is discussed in Chapter 14 on drug abuse and reward. The link of DAT occupancy to substance abuse is also discussed in Chapter 14. When 50% or more of DATs are occupied more slowly and in a more long-lasting manner, especially with controlled-release formulations, stimulants are less abusable and more useful for attention deficit hyperactivity disorder (ADHD), discussed in more detail in Chapter 12. The issue to be considered here is whether a low level of slow-onset and long-lasting DAT occupancy is the desirable solution for the DAT mechanism to be useful as an antidepressant: thus, not too much or too fast DAT inhibition and therefore abusable; not too little DAT inhibition and therefore ineffective; but just enough DAT inhibition with slow enough onset and long enough duration of action to make it an antidepressant.

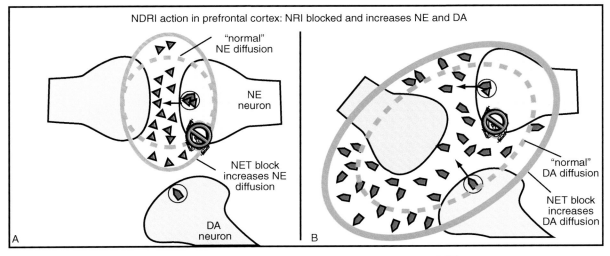

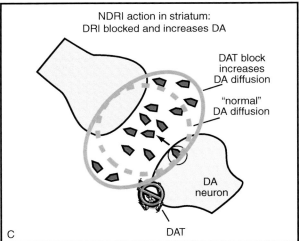

Figure 7-37. NDRI actions in prefrontal cortex and striatum. Norepinephrine–dopamine reuptake inhibitors (NDRIs) block the transporters for both norepinephrine (NET) and dopamine (DAT). (A) NET blockade in the prefrontal cortex leads to an increase in synaptic norepinephrine, thus increasing norepinephrine's diffusion radius. (B) Because the prefrontal cortex lacks DATs, and NETs transport dopamine as well as norepinephrine, NET blockade also leads to an increase in synaptic dopamine as well as NE in the prefrontal cortex, further increasing DA's diffusion radius. Thus, despite the absence of DAT in the prefrontal cortex, NDRIs still increase dopamine in the prefrontal cortex. (C) DAT is present in the striatum, and thus DAT inhibition increases dopamine diffusion there.

The fact that bupropion is not known to be particularly abusable, is not a scheduled substance, yet is proven effective for treating nicotine addiction, is consistent with the possibility that it is occupying DATs in the striatum and nucleus accumbens in a manner sufficient to mitigate craving but not sufficient to cause abuse (Figure 7-37C). This is discussed further in Chapter 14 on drug abuse and reward. Perhaps this is also how bupropion works in depression, combined with an equal action on NETs (Figure 7-37A and B). Clinical observations of depressed patients are also consistent with DAT and

NET inhibition as the mechanism of bupropion, since this agent appears especially useful in targeting the symptoms of "reduced positive affect" within the affective spectrum (see Figure 6-46), including improvement in the symptoms of loss of happiness, joy, interest, pleasure, energy, enthusiasm, alertness, and self-confidence.

Bupropion was originally marketed only in the US as an immediate-release dosage formulation with three-times-daily administration as an anti-depressant. Development of a twice-a-day formulation (bupropion SR) and more recently a once-a-day formulation (bupropion XL) have not only reduced the frequency of seizures at peak plasma drug levels, but have also increased convenience and enhanced compliance as well. Thus, the use of immediate-release bupropion is all but abandoned in favor of once-a-day administration. Now that bupropion SR and XL are generic in the US, some controversy exists over whether generic controlled-release technologies are as consistent as the original branded controlled-release technologies, and possibly might dose dump rather than deliver like the branded drugs, and be ineffective in some patients.

Bupropion is generally activating or even stimulating. Interestingly, bupropion does not appear to cause the bothersome sexual dysfunction that frequently occurs with antidepressants that act by SERT inhibition, probably because bupropion lacks a significant serotonergic component to its mechanism of action. Thus, bupropion has proven to be a useful antidepressant not only for patients who cannot tolerate the serotonergic side effects of SSRIs, but also for patients whose depression does not respond to serotonergic boosting by SSRIs. As discussed above, given its pharmacologic profile, bupropion is especially targeted at the symptoms of the "dopamine deficiency syndrome" and "reduced positive affect" (Figure 6-46). Almost every active clinician knows that patients who have residual symptoms of reduced positive affect following treatment with an SSRI or an SNRI, or who develop these symptoms as a side effect of an SSRI or SNRI, frequently benefit from switching to bupropion or from augmenting their SSRI or SNRI treatment with bupropion. The combination of bupropion with an SSRI or an SNRI has a theoretical rationale as a strategy for covering the entire symptom portfolio from symptoms of reduced positive affect to symptoms of increased negative affect (Figure 6-46).

Selective norepinephrine reuptake inhibitors (NRIs)

Although some tricyclic antidepressants (e.g., desipramine, maprotiline) block norepinephrine reuptake more potently than serotonin reuptake, even these tricyclics are not really selective, since they still block many other receptors such as α_1-adrenergic, H_1-histaminic, and muscarinic cholinergic receptors, as all tricyclics do. Tricyclic antidepressants are discussed later in this chapter.

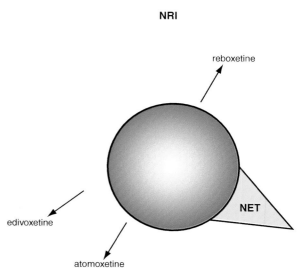

Figure 7-38. **Icon of a selective norepinephrine reuptake inhibitor.** Reboxetine, atomoxetine, and edivoxetine are antidepressants that have selective actions at the norepinephrine transporter (NET).

The first truly selective noradrenergic reuptake inhibitor marketed in Europe and other countries is reboxetine; the first in the US is atomoxetine (Figure 7-38). Both of these compounds are selective NRIs and lack the additional undesirable binding properties of tricyclic antidepressants. Reboxetine is approved as an antidepressant in Europe, but not in the US. Extensive testing in the US suggested inconsistent efficacy in major depression with the possibility of being less effective than SSRIs, so reboxetine was dropped from further development as an antidepressant in the US. Atomoxetine was never developed as an antidepressant but is marketed for the treatment of attention deficit hyperactivity disorder (ADHD) in the US and other countries. ADHD treatments are discussed in Chapter 12.

Many of the important concepts about NET inhibition have already been covered in the section on SNRIs above. This includes the observations that NET inhibition not only raises NE diffusely throughout all NE neuronal projections, but also raises DA levels in prefrontal cortex (Figure 7-34). It also includes both the therapeutic and side-effect profile of NET inhibition. There is some question about whether selective NET inhibition has any different clinical profile than when NET inhibition occurs simultaneously with SERT inhibition, such as when administering an SNRI or when giving a selective NRI with an SSRI. One thing that may be different is that NET inhibitors that are selective tend to be dosed so that there is a greater proportion of NET occupancy, close to saturation, compared to NET occupancy when dosed as an SNRI or as an NDRI, which as mentioned above may occupy substantially fewer NETs at clinically effective antidepressant doses. This higher degree of NET occupancy of selective NET inhibitors may be necessary for optimal efficacy for either depression or ADHD if there is no simultaneous SERT or DAT inhibition with which to add or synergize. One of the interesting observations is that high degrees of selective NET inhibition, although often activating, can also be sedating in some patients. Perhaps this is due to "over-tuning" noradrenergic input to cortical pyramidal neurons, which is discussed in Chapter 12 on ADHD.

There is less documentation that NET inhibition is as helpful for anxiety disorders as SERT inhibition, and neither of the selective NRIs discussed above is approved for anxiety disorders, although atomoxetine is approved for adult ADHD, which is frequently comorbid with anxiety disorders. A new selective NET inhibitor, sometimes called a NERI (norepinephrine reuptake inhibitor) and known as edivoxetine, is in testing as an augmenting agent to SSRIs in depression (Figure 7-38).

Agomelatine

Depression can alter circadian rhythms, causing a phase delay in the sleep/wake cycle (Figure 7-39). The degree of this phase delay correlates with the severity of depression. Numerous physiological measurements of circadian rhythms are also altered in depression, from flattening of the daily body temperature cycle to

elevation of cortisol secretion throughout the day, and also reducing the melatonin secretion that normally peaks at night and in the dark (Figure 7-40). Elevations of cortisol secretion and abnormalities of the HPA (hypothalamic–pituitary–adrenal) axis in depression are also discussed in Chapter 6 (see Figures 6-39A and 6-39B). Other normal circadian rhythms that may be disrupted in depression include a reduction in BDNF (brain-derived neurotrophic factor) and the neurogenesis that normally peaks at night (also discussed in Chapter 6: see Figures 6-36 through 6-38). Desynchronization of biological processes is so pervasive in depression that it is plausible to characterize depression as fundamentally a circadian illness. It is possible that depression is due to a "broken" circadian clock. Numerous genes operate in a circadian manner, sensitive to light–dark rhythms and called clock genes. Abnormalities in various clock genes have been linked to mood disorders. Also supporting the notion that depression is an illness with a broken circadian clock is the recent demonstration that specific pharmacological mechanisms – namely, melatonergic actions combined with monoaminergic actions – can resynchronize circadian rhythms in depression, essentially fixing the broken circadian clock and thereby exerting an antidepressant effect.

Agomelatine is an antidepressant approved in many countries outside of the US; it has agonist actions at melatonin 1 (MT_1) and melatonin 2 (MT_2) receptors and antagonist actions at $5HT_{2C}$ receptors (Figure 7-41). $5HT_{2C}$ antagonist actions are discussed in Chapter 5, and are a property of the antidepressants fluoxetine and mirtazapine and the atypical antipsychotics with antidepressant actions quetiapine and olanzapine. $5HT_{2C}$ receptors are not

Depression Causes Phase Delay in the Circadian Rhythms of Sleep-Wake Cycles

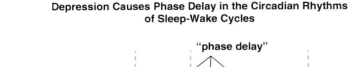

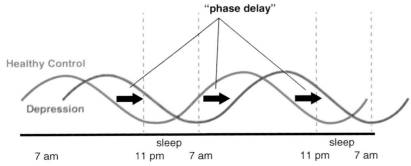

Figure 7-39. Depression causes phase delay in circadian rhythms of sleep/wake cycles. Circadian rhythms describe events that occur on a 24-hour cycle. Many biological systems follow a circadian rhythm; in particular, circadian rhythms are key to the regulation of sleep/wake cycles. In patients with depression, the circadian rhythm is often "phase delayed," which means that because wakefulness is not promoted in the morning, such patients tend to sleep later. They also have trouble falling asleep at night, which further promotes feelings of sleepiness during the day.

Physiological Measurements of Circadian Rhythms are Altered in Depression

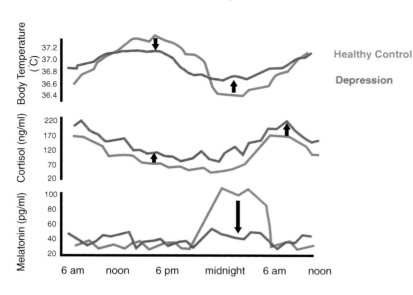

Healthy Control

Depression

Figure 7-40. Physiological measurements of circadian rhythms are altered in depression. Circadian rhythms are evident in multiple biological functions, including body temperature, hormone levels, blood pressure, metabolism, cellular regeneration, sleep/wake cycles, and DNA transcription and translation. The internal coordination ordered by the circadian rhythm is essential to optimal health. In depression, there are altered physiological measurements of circadian rhythms, including less fluctuation in body temperature over the course of a 24-hour cycle, the same pattern but elevated cortisol levels over 24 hours, and the absence of a spike in melatonin levels at night.

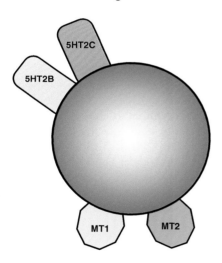

agomelatine

Figure 7-41. Agomelatine. Endogenous melatonin is secreted by the pineal gland and mainly acts in the suprachiasmatic nucleus to regulate circadian rhythms. There are three types of receptors for melatonin: MT_1 and MT_2, which are both involved in sleep, and MT_3, which is actually the enzyme NRH:quinine oxidoreductase 2 and not thought to be involved in sleep physiology. Agomelatine is not only an MT_1 and MT_2 receptor agonist, but is also a $5HT_{2C}$ and $5HT_{2B}$ receptor antagonist and is available as an antidepressant in Europe.

only located in the midbrain raphe and prefrontal cortex where they regulate the release of dopamine and norepinephrine (see Figures 5-52A and 5-52B); $5HT_{2C}$ receptors are also localized in the

suprachiasmatic nucleus (SCN) of the hypothalamus, the brain's "pacemaker," where they interact with melatonin receptors (Figures 7-42A through 7-42D). Light is detected by the retina during the day, and this information travels to the SCN via the retinohypothalamic tract (Figure 7-42A), which normally synchronizes many circadian rhythms downstream from the SCN. For example, both melatonin receptors and $5HT_{2C}$ receptors fluctuate in a circadian manner in the SCN, with high receptor expression at night/dark and low receptor expression in the day/light. That makes sense, since melatonin is only secreted at night in the dark (Figure 7-42B). In depression, however, circadian rhythms are "out of synch" including low melatonin secretion at night among numerous other changes (Figures 7-39, 7-40, 7-42C). Agomelatine, by stimulating melatonin receptors in the SCN and simultaneously blocking $5HT_{2C}$ receptors there as well, appears to resynchronize circadian rhythms, reverse the phase delay of depression, and thereby exert an antidepressant effect (Figure 7-42D).

Melatonergic actions are not sufficient for this antidepressant effect, as melatonin itself and selective melatonergic MT_1 and MT_2 receptor agonists do not have proven antidepressant action. $5HT_{2C}$ antagonism has been shown to interact with melatonin MT_1/MT_2 agonism by affecting the secretion of melatonin by the pineal gland, especially by regulating the suppression of melatonin secretion by light. The combination of $5HT_{2C}$ antagonism plus MT_1/MT_2 agonism creates numerous

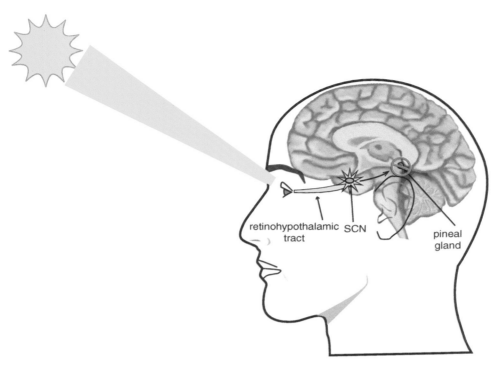

Figure 7-42A. The setting of circadian rhythms, part 1. Although various factors can affect the setting of circadian rhythms, light is the most powerful synchronizer. When light enters through the eye it is translated via the retinohypothalamic tract to the suprachiasmatic nucleus (or SCN) within the hypothalamus. The SCN, in turn, signals the pineal gland to turn off melatonin production.

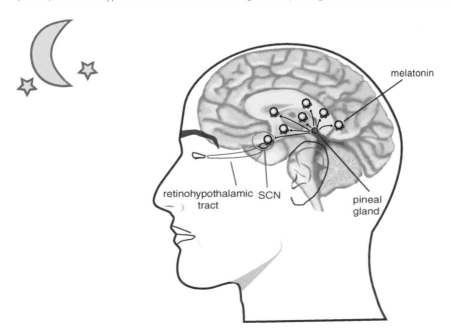

Figure 7-42B. The setting of circadian rhythms, part 2. During darkness, there is no input from the retinohypothalamic tract to the suprachiasmatic nucleus (SCN) within the hypothalamus. Thus, darkness signals the pineal gland to produce melatonin. Melatonin, in turn, can act on the SCN to reset circadian rhythms.

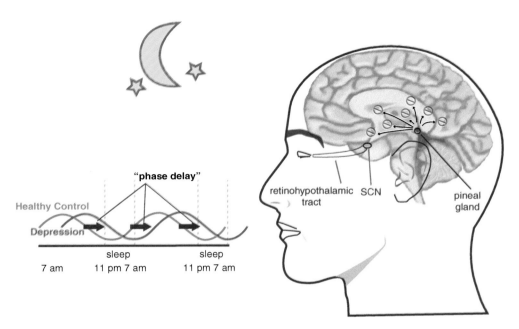

Figure 7-42C. The setting of circadian rhythms, part 3. In patients with depression, circadian rhythms are often "phase delayed," which means that because wakefulness is not promoted in the morning, such patients tend to sleep later. They also have trouble falling asleep at night, which further promotes feelings of sleepiness during the day. The phase delay observed in depression may be related to the fact that, even in darkness, there seems to be lack of melatonin production in the brains of patients with depression.

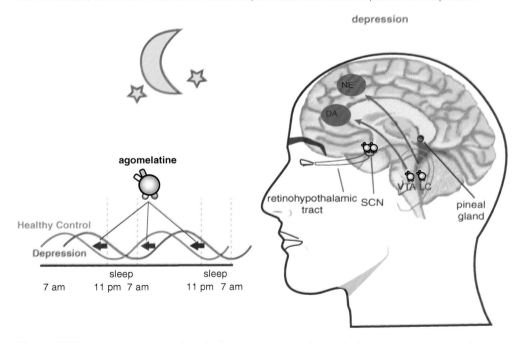

Figure 7-42D. The setting of circadian rhythms, part 4. Agomelatine, which acts as an agonist at melatonin 1 and 2 receptors, may resynchronize circadian rhythms by acting as "substitute melatonin." Thus, even in the absence of melatonin production in the pineal gland, agomelatine can bind to melatonin 1 and 2 receptors in the suprachiasmatic nucleus (SCN) to reset circadian rhythms. In addition, by blocking serotonin 2C receptors in the ventral tegmental area (VTA) and locus coeruleus (LC), agomelatine promotes dopamine (DA) and norepinephrine (NE) release in the prefrontal cortex (see Figures 5-52A, 5-52B, 7-43).

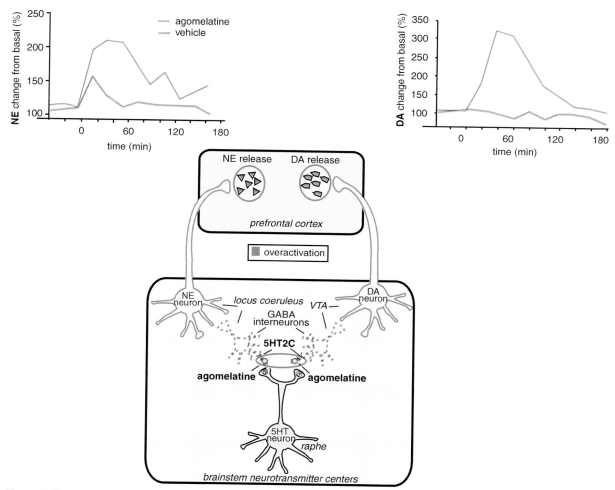

Figure 7-43. Agomelatine releases norepinephrine and dopamine in the prefrontal cortex. Normally, serotonin binding at $5HT_{2C}$ receptors on γ-aminobutyric acid (GABA) interneurons in the brainstem inhibits norepinephrine and dopamine release in the prefrontal cortex. When a $5HT_{2C}$ antagonist such as agomelatine binds to $5HT_{2C}$ receptors on GABA interneurons (bottom red circle), it prevents serotonin from binding there and thus prevents inhibition of norepinephrine and dopamine release in the prefrontal cortex; in other words, it disinhibits their release (top red circles).

biological effects that are not triggered by either mechanism alone: namely, enhancing neurogenesis and BDNF; resetting sleep/wake and dark/light phases; decreasing stress-induced glutamate release; regulating downstream signal transduction cascades and clock genes; resynchronizing circadian rhythms and, most critically, antidepressant actions. Not only does $5HT_{2C}$ antagonism raise norepinephrine and dopamine in prefrontal cortex, but with simultaneous stimulation of MT_1 and MT_2 receptors, agomelatine apparently resynchronizes circadian rhythms which potentially can optimize these changes in monoamines (Figure 7-43).

Alpha-2 antagonist actions and mirtazapine

Alpha-2 (α_2) antagonism is another way to enhance the release of monoamines and exert an antidepressant action. Recall that norepinephrine turns off its own release by interacting with presynaptic α_2 autoreceptors on noradrenergic neurons, as discussed in

Chapter 6 and illustrated in Figures 6-28 and 6-29. Therefore, when an α_2 antagonist is administered, norepinephrine can no longer turn off its own release and noradrenergic neurons are thus disinhibited from their axon terminals, such as those in the raphe and in the cortex (Figure 7-44A).

Recall also that norepinephrine turns off serotonin release by interacting with presynaptic α_2 heteroreceptors on serotonergic neurons (Figure 6-30C). Alpha-2 antagonists block norepinephrine from turning off serotonin release because α_2 heteroreceptors on serotonin axon terminals are blocked even in the presence of norepinephrine (Figure 7-44B). Therefore, serotonergic neurons become disinhibited and serotonin release is enhanced (Figure 7-44B). It is as though α_2 antagonists acting at serotonin axon terminals "cut the brake cable" of noradrenergic inhibition (NE stepping on the brake to prevent 5HT release, shown in Figure 6-30C, is blocked in Figure 7-44B).

A second mechanism to increase serotonin release after an α_2 antagonist is administered may be even more important. Recall that norepinephrine neurons from the locus coeruleus innervate the cell bodies of serotonergic neurons in the midbrain raphe and stimulate serotonin release from serotonin axon terminals via a postsynaptic α_1 receptor on the serotonin cell body (Figure 6-30B). Thus, when α_2 antagonists cause norepinephrine release in the raphe (Figure 7-44A, box 2), this also causes stimulation of postsynaptic α_1 receptors on serotonin neuronal cell bodies in the raphe (Figure 7-44B, box 2), thereby provoking more serotonin release from the downstream axon terminals, such as those in the cortex shown in Figure 7-44C box 1. This is like stepping on the serotonin accelerator. Thus, α_2 antagonists both "cut the brake cable" (Figure 7-44B) and "step on the accelerator" (Figure 7-44C) to facilitate serotonin release. Alpha-2 antagonist actions therefore yield dual enhancement of both 5HT and NE release, but unlike SNRIs they have this effect by a mechanism independent of blockade of monoamine transporters. These two mechanisms, monoamine transport blockade and α_2 antagonism, are synergistic, so that blocking them simultaneously gives a much more powerful disinhibitory signal to these two neurotransmitters than if only one mechanism is blocked. For this reason, the α_2 antagonist mirtazapine is often combined with SNRIs for treatment of cases that do not respond to an SNRI alone. This combination is sometimes called "California rocket fuel" because of the potentially powerful antidepressant action blasting the patient out of the depths of depression.

Although no selective α_2 antagonist is available for use as an antidepressant, there are several drugs with prominent α_2 properties, including mirtazapine, mianserin, and some of the atypical antipsychotics discussed in Chapter 5 (see Figure 5-37). Mirtazapine does not block any monoamine transporter; however, it not only blocks α_2 receptors, but has additional potent antagonist actions upon $5HT_{2A}$ receptors, $5HT_{2C}$ receptors, $5HT_3$ receptors, and H_1 histamine receptors (Figure 7-45). Two other α_2 antagonists are marketed as antidepressants in some countries (but not the US), namely mianserin (worldwide except US) and setiptiline (Japan). Unlike mirtazapine, mianserin also has potent α_1 antagonist properties which tend to mitigate its ability to enhance serotonergic neurotransmission, so that this drug enhances predominantly noradrenergic neurotransmission, yet with associated $5HT_{2A}$, $5HT_{2C}$, $5HT_3$, and H_1 antagonist properties (Figure 7-45).

$5HT_{2C}$ antagonist action as a potential antidepressant mechanism has been discussed above in regard to agomelatine and also in Chapter 5, and should theoretically contribute to the antidepressant effects of mirtazapine and mianserin as well. The H_1 antihistaminic actions of mirtazapine and mianserin (Figure 7-45) should theoretically relieve insomnia at night, and improve anxiety during the day, but could also cause drowsiness during the day. Combined with the $5HT_{2C}$ antagonist properties described above, the H_1 antihistaminic actions of mirtazapine could also cause weight gain (Figure 7-45).

5HT₃ antagonist action

$5HT_3$ receptors are localized in the chemoreceptor trigger zone of the brainstem, where they mediate nausea and vomiting, and in the gastrointestinal tract, where they mediate nausea, vomiting, and diarrhea/bowel motility when stimulated. Blocking these receptors can therefore protect against serotonin-induced gastrointestinal side effects that often accompany agents that increase 5HT release.

$5HT_3$ receptors in the brain also regulate the release of various neurotransmitters, especially norepinephrine and acetylcholine (Figure 7-46A), but also possibly serotonin, dopamine, and histamine as well. Serotonin acting at $5HT_3$ receptors reduces the release of these neurotransmitters (Figure 7-46B), so blocking $5HT_3$ receptors causes disinhibition of these

Alpha-2 Antagonism Increases NE Release in Raphe and Cortex

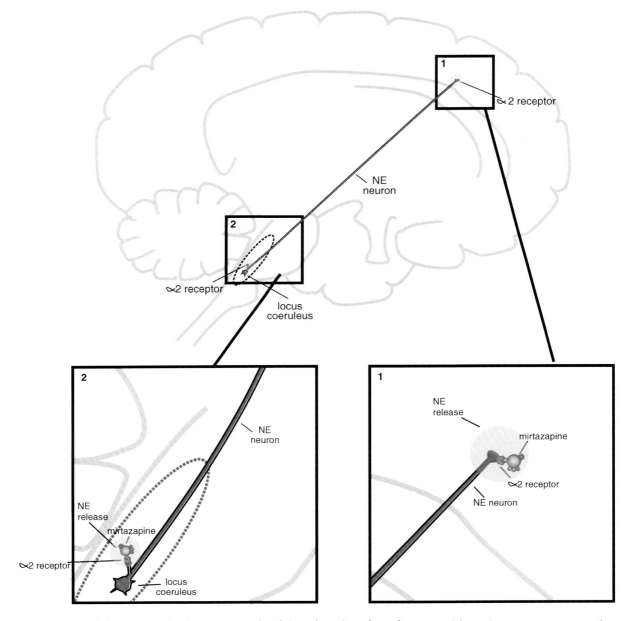

Figure 7-44A. Alpha-2 antagonism increases norepinephrine release in raphe and cortex. α_2-Adrenergic receptors are presynaptic autoreceptors and thus are the "brakes" on noradrenergic neurons. An α_2 antagonist (e.g., mirtazapine) can therefore increase norepinephrine release by binding to these receptors in the locus coeruleus (2) and in the cortex (1).

Alpha-2 Antagonism Increases 5HT and NE Release in Cortex

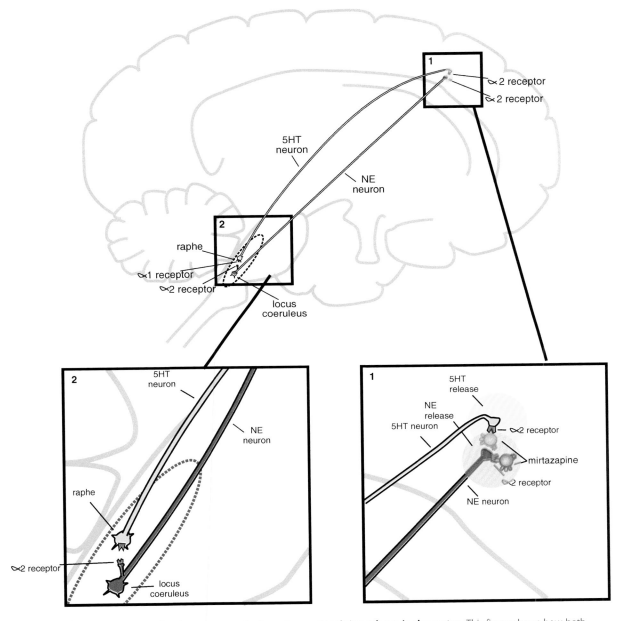

Figure 7-44B. Alpha-2 antagonism increases serotonin and norepinephrine release in the cortex. This figure shows how both noradrenergic and serotonergic neurotransmission are enhanced by α₂ antagonists. The noradrenergic neuron is disinhibited in the cortex because an α₂ antagonist is blocking its presynaptic α₂ autoreceptors. This has the effect of "cutting the brake cables" for norepinephrine (NE) release. In addition, α₂ antagonists "cut the 5HT brake cable" when α₂ presynaptic heteroreceptors are blocked on the 5HT axon terminal, thus leading to enhanced serotonin release.

Alpha-2 Antagonism in Raphe Stimulates 5HT Release in Cortex

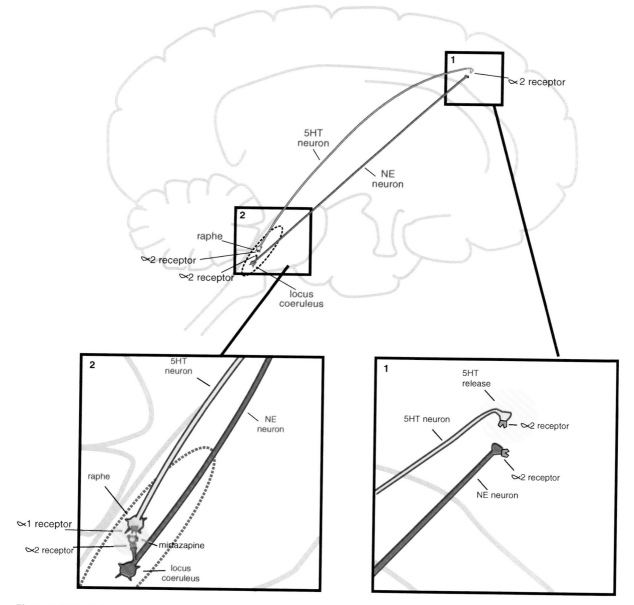

Figure 7-44C. Alpha-2 antagonism in raphe stimulates serotonin release in cortex. The noradrenergic neuron is disinhibited at its axon terminals in the brainstem because an α_2 antagonist is blocking its presynaptic α_2 autoreceptors (2). This has the effect of "cutting the brake cables" for norepinephrine (NE) release. Norepinephrine can then stimulate α_1 receptors on the serotonergic neuron, leading to serotonin release in the cortex (1).

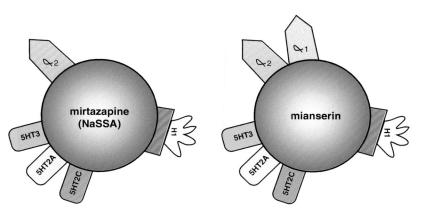

Figure 7-45. Mirtazapine and mianserin. Mirtazapine is sometimes called a noradrenergic and specific serotonergic antidepressant (NaSSA). Its primary therapeutic action is α_2 antagonism, as shown in Figures 7-44A through 7-44C. It also blocks three serotonin (5HT) receptors: $5HT_{2A}$, $5HT_{2C}$, and $5HT_3$. Finally, it blocks histamine 1 (H_1) receptors. Mianserin is also a NaSSA and has a similar binding profile to mirtazapine, the only difference being additional effects at α_1 receptors.

same neurotransmitters and thus enhances their release (Figure 7-46C). Thus, agents such as mirtazapine with $5HT_3$ antagonist properties should enhance the release of various neurotransmitters and this could contribute to antidepressant actions. Mianserin has $5HT_3$ antagonist properties, and so do some atypical antipsychotics. Potent $5HT_3$ antagonism is also one of the five multimodal pharmacologic actions of an experimental antidepressant vortioxetine, in late-stage clinical trials.

Serotonin antagonist/reuptake inhibitors (SARIs)

The prototype drug that blocks serotonin 2A and 2C ($5HT_{2A}$ and $5HT_{2C}$) receptors as well as serotonin reuptake is trazodone, classified as a serotonin antagonist/reuptake inhibitor (SARI), or, more fully, as a serotonin 2A/2C antagonist and serotonin reuptake inhibitor (Figure 7-47). Nefazodone is another SARI with robust $5HT_{2A}$ antagonist actions and weaker $5HT_{2C}$ antagonist and SERT inhibition, but is no longer commonly used because of rare liver toxicity (Figure 7-47). Trazodone is a very interesting agent, since it acts like two different drugs, depending upon the dose and the formulation. We discussed a very similar situation in Chapter 5 for quetiapine, and illustrated this in Figures 5-47 through 5-50.

Different drug at different doses?

The combined actions of $5HT_{2A}/5HT_{2C}$ antagonism with SERT inhibition only occur at moderate to high doses of trazodone (Figure 7-48). Doses of trazodone lower than those effective for antidepressant action are frequently used for the effective treatment of insomnia. Low doses exploit trazodone's potent actions as a $5HT_{2A}$ antagonist, and also its properties as an antagonist of H_1-histaminic and α_1-adrenergic receptors, but do not adequately exploit its SERT or $5HT_{2C}$ inhibition properties, which are weaker (Figure 7-48). As discussed in Chapter 5 and illustrated in Figure 5-38, blocking the brain's arousal system with H_1 and α_1 antagonism can cause sedation or sleep, and along with $5HT_{2A}$ antagonist properties this may explain the mechanism of how low doses of trazodone work as a hypnotic (Figure 7-48). Since insomnia is one of the most frequent residual symptoms of depression after treatment with an SSRI (discussed earlier in this chapter and illustrated in Figure 7-5), a hypnotic is often necessary for patients with a major depressive episode. Not only can a hypnotic potentially relieve the insomnia itself, but treating insomnia in patients with major depression may also increase remission rates due to improvement of other symptoms such as loss of energy and depressed mood. This may be the case not only for low-dose trazodone but also for the combination of antidepressants with sedative hypnotics (such as eszopiclone and others) in general, as long as insomnia is relieved. Thus, the ability of low doses of trazodone to improve sleep in depressed patients may be an important mechanism whereby trazodone can augment the efficacy of other antidepressants.

Trazodone inhibits $5HT_{2A}$ receptors at essentially any clinical dose, but to get an antidepressant action the dose must be raised to recruit SERT inhibition and thus to raise serotonin levels (Figure 7-48). However, what happens when trazodone raises serotonin levels is different than what happens when an SSRI/SNRI does this. Namely, the SSRI/SNRI raises

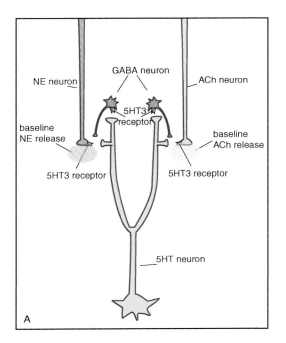

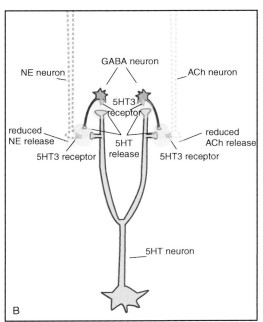

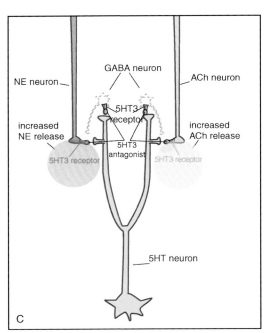

Figure 7-46. 5HT₃ antagonists increase norepinephrine and acetylcholine release. (A) Serotonergic neurons synapse with noradrenergic neurons, cholinergic neurons, and GABAergic interneurons, all of which contain serotonin 3 (5HT₃) receptors. (B) When serotonin is released, it binds to 5HT₃ receptors on GABAergic neurons, which release GABA onto noradrenergic and cholinergic neurons, thus reducing release of norepinephrine (NE) and acetylcholine (ACh), respectively. In addition, serotonin may bind to 5HT₃ receptors on noradrenergic and cholinergic neurons, further reducing release of those neurotransmitters. (C) A 5HT₃ antagonist binding at GABAergic neurons inhibits GABA release, which in turn disinhibits (or turns on) noradrenergic and cholinergic neurons, leading to release of norepinephrine and acetylcholine, respectively. Likewise, a 5HT₃ antagonist binding directly at noradrenergic and cholinergic neurons prevents serotonin from binding there and inhibiting release of their neurotransmitters.

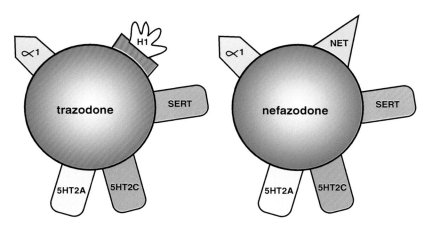

Figure 7-47. Serotonin antagonist/reuptake inhibitors. Shown here are icons for two serotonin 2A ($5HT_{2A}$) antagonist/reuptake inhibitors (SARIs): trazodone and nefazodone. These agents have a dual action, but the two mechanisms are different from the dual action of the serotonin–norepinephrine reuptake inhibitors (SNRIs). The SARIs act by potent blockade of $5HT_{2A}$ receptors as well as dose-dependent blockade of $5HT_{2C}$ receptors and the serotonin transporter (SRI). SARIs also block a_1-adrenergic receptors. In addition, trazodone has the unique property of histamine 1 (H_1) receptor antagonism and nefazodone has the unique property of norepinephrine reuptake inhibition (NRI).

Trazodone as an Antidepressant:
Serotonin Antagonist/Reuptake Inhibitor (SARI)

Trazodone as a Hypnotic:
Multifunctional Neurotransmitter Antagonist

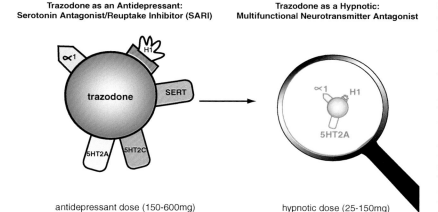

antidepressant dose (150-600mg)

hypnotic dose (25-150mg)

Figure 7-48. Trazodone at different doses. High doses that recruit saturation of the serotonin transporter (i.e., 150–600 mg) are required for trazodone to have antidepressant actions (icon on left). At this high antidepressant dose, trazodone is a multifunctional serotonergic agent with antagonist actions at $5HT_{2A}$ and $5HT_{2C}$ receptors as well. Thus, its antidepressant actions are attributed to these serotonergic properties. Trazodone is also an a_1 and H_1 antagonist at these doses. At lower doses of trazodone (i.e., 25–150 mg), it does not saturate the serotonin transporter; thus it loses its antidepressant actions while retaining antagonist actions at $5HT_{2A}$, a_1, and H_1 receptors, and corresponding hypnotic efficacy (icon on right). Relative selectivities of trazodone for four key binding sites are shown in the chart at the bottom of the figure.

Relative Selectivities of Trazodone at Different Doses

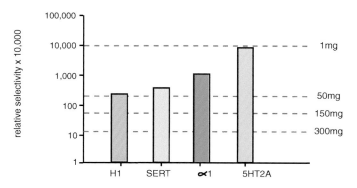

SSRI Action

SARI Action at 5HT Synapses

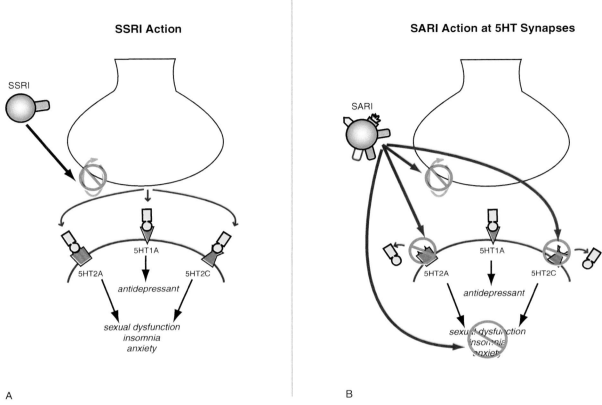

Figure 7-49. SSRI versus SARI. (A) Inhibition of the serotonin transporter (SERT) by a selective serotonin reuptake inhibitor (SSRI) at the presynaptic neuron increases serotonin at all receptors, with 5HT$_{1A}$-mediated antidepressant actions but also 5HT$_{2A}$- and 5HT$_{2C}$-mediated sexual dysfunction, insomnia, and anxiety. (B) SERT inhibition by a serotonin 2A (5HT$_{2A}$) antagonist/reuptake inhibitor (SARI) at the presynaptic neuron increases serotonin at 5HT$_{1A}$ receptors, where it leads to antidepressant actions. However, SARI action also blocks serotonin actions at 5HT$_{2A}$ and 5HT$_{2C}$ receptors, thus failing to cause sexual dysfunction, insomnia, or anxiety. In fact, these blocking actions at 5HT$_{2A}$ and 5HT$_{2C}$ receptors can improve insomnia and anxiety, and theoretically can exert antidepressant actions of their own.

serotonin levels to act at all serotonin receptors, both theoretically with therapeutic actions by stimulating 5HT$_{1A}$ receptors, and with side effects as the "cost of doing business" by concomitantly stimulating 5HT$_{2A}$ and 5HT$_{2C}$ receptors that theoretically cause sexual dysfunction, insomnia, and activation/anxiety, as well as other 5HT receptors (Figure 7-49A). However, with trazodone, 5HT$_{1A}$ receptors are stimulated by rising serotonin levels when SERT is inhibited, but 5HT$_{2A}$ and 5HT$_{2C}$ receptors are blocked by trazodone (Figure 7-49B). This pharmacologic profile alters the clinical profile of trazodone, and explains why trazodone is not associated with sexual dysfunction or insomnia/anxiety and is in fact a treatment for insomnia/anxiety. The same clinical

profile applies to other agents with 5HT$_{2A}$ antagonist properties such as atypical antipsychotics and mirtazapine, when added to SSRIs/SNRIs, which changes the clinical profile of SSRIs/SNRIs given as monotherapies (Figure 7-49). Also, the combination of 5HT$_{2A}$ antagonism with 5HT$_{1A}$ stimulation causes enhancement of both glutamate and dopamine release downstream, as discussed in Chapter 5 and illustrated in Figures 5-15 and 5-16, which may also contribute to the antidepressant profile of agents that simultaneously block 5HT$_{2A}$ receptors and stimulate 5HT$_{1A}$ receptors, such as trazodone, mirtazapine, some atypical antipsychotics, and the combination of SSRIs/SNRIs with these various drugs that are 5HT$_{2A}$ antagonists.

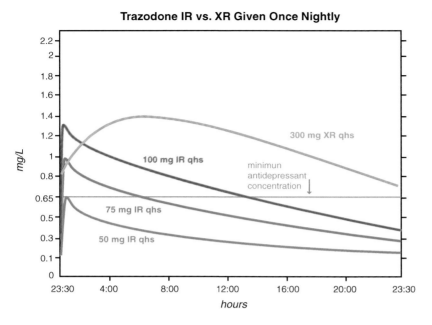

Trazodone IR vs. XR Given Once Nightly

Figure 7-50. Trazodone IR versus XR given once nightly. Shown here are steady-state estimates of the plasma trazodone levels from the hypnotic dosing of 50, 75, or 100 mg once nightly of trazodone immediate-release (IR) over 9 days. Peak drug concentrations are reached rapidly with a similarly rapid fall-off over night. The minimum levels estimated for antidepressant actions of trazodone are reached transiently, if at all, by hypnotic dosing. By contrast, 300 mg of trazodone extended-release (XR) given once nightly generates plasma levels that rise slowly and never fall below minimum antidepressant concentrations. Peak levels of trazodone XR at 300 mg are about the same as the peak levels of trazodone IR at 100 mg.

Different drug in different formulations?

Trazodone is not commonly used at high doses as an antidepressant because it has a short half-life requiring multiple daily doses, and can be very sedating at antidepressant dosing levels. Trazodone comes in an immediate-release (IR) formulation and in various controlled-release formulations in different countries (Figure 7-50). The immediate-release formulation of trazodone has a relatively rapid onset and short duration of action, and in low doses as a hypnotic, patients only need to take it once a day at night (Figure 7-50). Trazodone levels rise rapidly and then fall from their peaks quickly after causing peak dose sedation, making the hypnotic actions rapid in onset, but wearing off before morning so there is no hangover effect (Figure 7-50). These pharmacologic properties make trazodone at low doses an ideal hypnotic but not an ideal antidepressant.

At higher antidepressant doses administered once a day at night, there can be a hangover effect the next morning; splitting the antidepressant dose into two or three times a day still leads to accumulation of trazodone levels and unacceptable daytime sedation (Figure 7-50). By contrast, high doses of controlled-release formulations given once daily at night do not attain the sedating peak levels of the immediate-release during the day, and thus are antidepressant without sedation, which is ideal for an antidepressant (Figure 7-50). For unclear reasons, high-dose trazodone in controlled-release formulations is not as extensively used in clinical practice as is the combination of low-dose trazodone with SSRIs/SNRIs, which is pharmacologically similar. Perhaps clinicians are not aware that the additional properties of trazodone added to SSRIs/SNRIs are likely not only to boost the efficacy of SSRIs/SNRIs in depression and anxiety, but also to have more than a hypnotic effect. These therapeutic effects might also be possible with the more tolerable controlled-release formulations of trazodone as a high-dose monotherapy.

Classic antidepressants: MAO inhibitors

The first clinically effective antidepressants to be discovered were inhibitors of the enzyme monoamine oxidase (MAO). They were discovered by accident when an anti-tuberculosis drug was observed to help depression that coexisted in some of the patients who had tuberculosis. This anti-tuberculosis drug, iproniazid, was eventually found to work in depression by inhibiting the enzyme MAO. However, inhibition of MAO was unrelated to its anti-tubercular actions. Although best known as powerful antidepressants, the monoamine oxidase inhibitors (MAOIs) are also highly effective therapeutic agents for certain anxiety disorders such as panic disorder and social phobia. MAOIs tend to be under-utilized in clinical practice, both because of the availability of many other options, and because of several prevailing myths and misinformation about MAOIs that prevent most modern-day clinicians from gaining familiarity with them.

The MAOIs phenelzine, tranylcypromine, and isocarboxazid are all irreversible enzyme inhibitors, and thus enzyme activity returns only after new enzyme is synthesized about 2–3 weeks later. Amphetamine is also a weak but reversible MAO inhibitor, and some MAOIs have properties related to amphetamine. For example, tranylcypromine has a chemical structure modeled on amphetamine, and thus in addition to MAO inhibitor properties, also has amphetamine-like dopamine-releasing properties. The MAOI selegiline itself does not have amphetamine-like properties, but is metabolized to both *l*-amphetamine and *l*-methamphetamine. Thus, there is a close mechanistic link between some MAOIs and additional amphetamine-like dopamine-releasing actions. It is therefore not surprising that one of the augmenting agents utilized to boost MAOIs in treatment-resistant patients is amphetamine, administered by experts with great caution while monitoring blood pressure.

MAO subtypes

MAO exists in two subtypes, A and B (Table 7-1). The A form preferentially metabolizes the monoamines most closely linked to depression (i.e., serotonin and norepinephrine) whereas the B form preferentially metabolizes trace amines such as phenylethylamine. Both MAO-A and MAO-B metabolize dopamine and tyramine. Both MAO-A and MAO-B are found in the brain. Noradrenergic neurons (Figure 6-26) and dopaminergic neurons (Figure 4-6) are thought to contain both MAO-A and MAO-B, with perhaps MAO-A activity predominant, whereas serotonergic neurons are thought to contain only MAO-B (Figure 5-14). MAO-A is the major form of this enzyme outside of the brain, with the exception of platelets and lymphocytes, which have MAO-B (Table 7-1).

Brain MAO-A must be inhibited for antidepressant efficacy to occur with MAOI treatment (Figure 7-51). This is not surprising, since this is the form of MAO that preferentially metabolizes serotonin and norepinephrine, two of the three monoamines linked to depression and to antidepressant actions, both of which demonstrate increased brain levels after MAO-A inhibition (Figure 7-51). MAO-A, along with MAO-B, also metabolizes dopamine, but inhibition of MAO-A alone does not appear to lead to robust increases in brain dopamine levels, since MAO-B can still metabolize dopamine (Figure 7-51).

Inhibition of MAO-B is not effective as an antidepressant, as there is no direct effect on either serotonin or norephinephrine metabolism, and little or no dopamine accumulates due to the continued action of MAO-A (Figure 7-52). What therefore is the therapeutic value of MAO-B inhibition? When this enzyme is selectively inhibited, it can boost the action of concomitantly administered levodopa in Parkinson's disease. MAO-B is also thought to convert some environmentally derived amine substrates, called protoxins, into toxins that may cause damage to neurons and possibly contribute to the cause or decline of function in Parkinson's disease. Inhibiting MAO-B could theoretically halt this process, and there is speculation that this might slow the degenerative course of various neurodegenerative disorders including Parkinson's disease, but this has not been proven. Two MAOIs, selegiline and rasagiline, when administered orally in doses selective for inhibition of MAO-B, are approved for use in patients with Parkinson's disease, but are not effective at these selective MAO-B doses as antidepressants.

When MAO-B is inhibited simultaneously with MAO-A, there is robust elevation of dopamine as well as serotonin and norepinephrine (Figure 7-53). This would theoretically provide the most powerful

Table 7-1 MAO subtypes

	MAO-A	MAO-B
Substrates	Serotonin Norepinephrine Dopamine Tyramine	Dopamine Tyramine Phenylethylamine
Tissue distribution	Brain, gut, liver, placenta, skin	Brain, platelets, lymphocytes

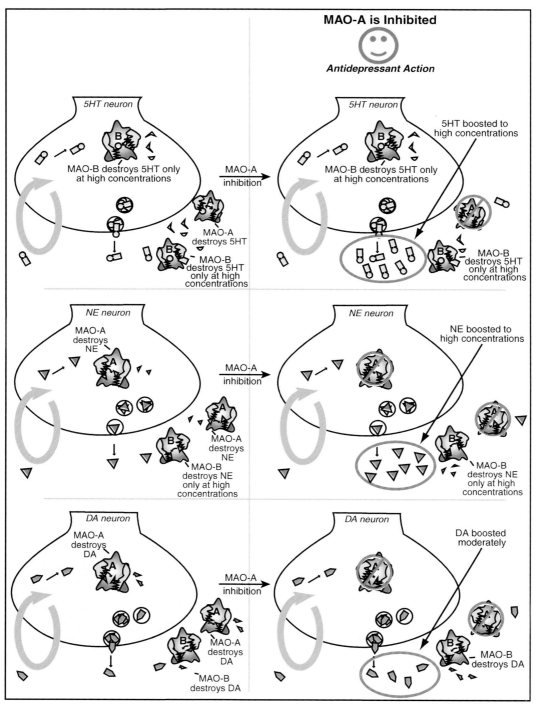

Figure 7-51. Monoamine oxidase A (MAO-A) inhibition. The enzyme MAO-A metabolizes serotonin (5HT) and norepinephrine (NE) as well as dopamine (DA) (left panels). Monoamine oxidase B (MAO-B) also metabolizes DA, but it metabolizes 5HT and NE only at high concentrations (left panels). This means that MAO-A inhibition increases 5HT, NE, and DA (right panels) but that the increase in DA is not as great as that of 5HT and NE because MAO-B can continue to destroy DA (bottom right panel). Inhibition of MAO-A is an efficacious antidepressant strategy.

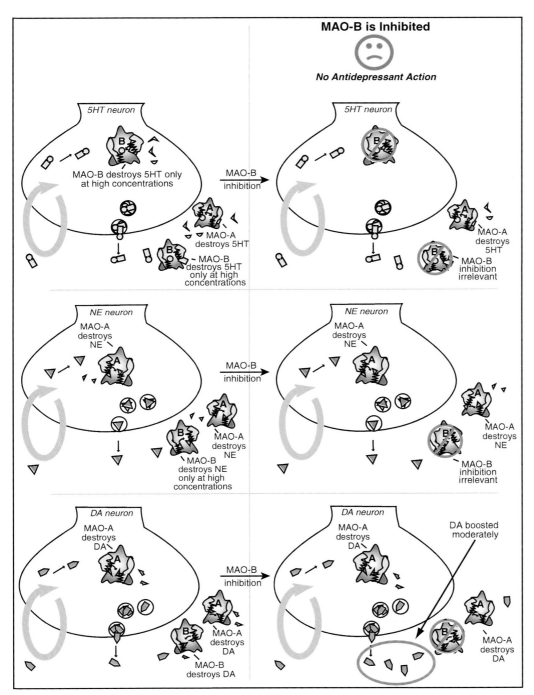

Figure 7-52. Monoamine oxidase B (MAO-B) inhibition. Selective inhibitors of MAO-B do not have antidepressant efficacy. This is because MAO-B metabolizes serotonin (5HT) and norepinephrine (NE) only at high concentrations (top two left panels). Since MAO-B's role in destroying 5HT and NE is small, its inhibition is not likely to be relevant to the concentrations of these neurotransmitters (top two right panels). Selective inhibition of MAO-B also has somewhat limited effects on dopamine (DA) concentrations, because MAO-A continues to destroy DA. However, inhibition of MAO-B does increase DA to some extent, which can be therapeutic in other disease states, such as Parkinson's disease.

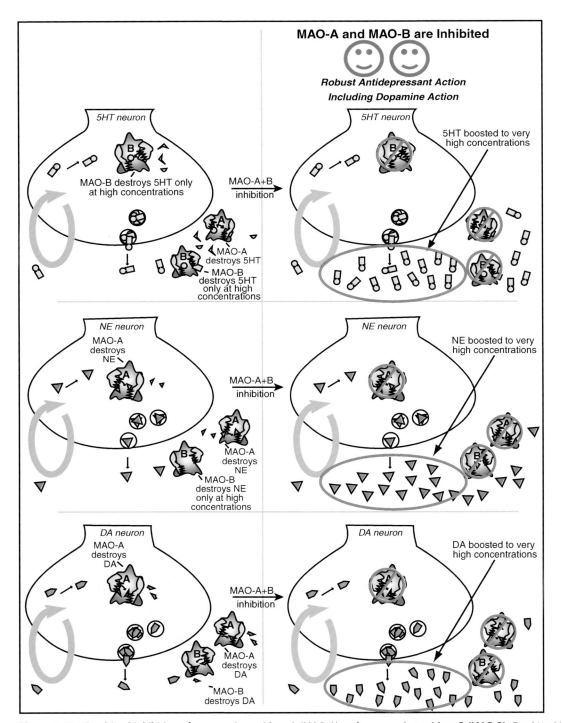

Figure 7-53. Combined inhibition of monoamine oxidase A (MAO-A) and monoamine oxidase B (MAO-B). Combined inhibition of MAO-A and MAO-B may have robust antidepressant actions owing to increases not only in serotonin (5HT) and norepinephrine (NE) but also dopamine (DA). Inhibition of both MAO-A, which metabolizes 5HT, NE, and DA, and MAO-B, which metabolizes primarily DA (left panels), leads to greater increases in each of these neurotransmitters than inhibition of either enzyme alone.

antidepressant efficacy across the range of depressive symptoms, from diminished positive affect to increased negative affect (Figure 6-46). Thus, MAO-A plus MAO-B inhibition is one of the few therapeutic strategies available to increase dopamine in depression, and therefore to treat refractory symptoms of diminished positive affect. This is a good reason for specialists in psychopharmacology to become adept at administering MAOIs, so that they can have an additional strategy within their armamentarium for cases with treatment-resistant symptoms of diminished positive affect, a very common problem in a referral practice.

Is increased MAO-A activity the cause of monoamine deficiency in some patients with depression?

One hypothesis for low levels of monoamines in depression comes from recent brain imaging studies of MAO-A, showing elevated levels of MAO-A activity in depressed patients. This would be predicted to lower the functional availability of monoamine neurotransmitters. MAO-A levels are not decreased by SSRIs, but of course are decreased by MAOIs. Some studies suggest that patients who recover from their depression with SSRI treatment, but do not simultaneously recover normal levels of MAO-A, have continuing vulnerability to relapse. Treatment with MAO-A inhibitors of course will uniquely lower the elevations in MAO-A activity compared to any other antidepressant, and thus may be preferable for some patients with depression. It is even possible that high levels of MAO-A may be linked to some types of treatment resistance. Supporting the potential role of abnormal MAO-A activity as a potential cause of depression or of some forms of treatment resistance is the discovery of a protein called R1 (repressor 1) that controls the expression of MAO-A. R1 may be depleted in both treated and untreated depression, causing a lack of repression of MAO-A synthesis and thus an increase in MAO-A activity in depression, with consequential decrease in monoamines. It is not currently possible to identify in advance those patients who might benefit from MAOI treatment, and these tests are not yet available in clinical practice, but it does point to the potential importance of knowing how to use MAOIs for the treatment of depression.

Myths, misinformation, and a manual for MAOIs

To prescribe MAOIs in clinical practice, it is necessary to understand how to manage two issues: diet and drug interactions. A series of tables that follows organizes these issues into several charts that address myths and misinformation about MAOIs, providing the truth about these myths and proposing clinical management solutions that we will call your MAOI "owner's manual."

The dietary tyramine interaction

One of the biggest barriers to using MAOIs has traditionally been the concern that a patient taking one of these drugs may develop a hypertensive crisis (Table 7-2) after ingesting tyramine in the diet. Normally, the release of norepinephrine by tyramine is inconsequential because MAO-A safely destroys this released norepinephrine (Figure 7-54). However, tyramine in the presence of MAO-A inhibition can elevate blood pressure because norepinephrine is not safely destroyed (Figure 7-55). The body normally has a huge capacity for processing tyramine, and the average person is able to handle approximately 400 mg of ingested tyramine before blood pressure is elevated. A so-called "high-tyramine diet" is unlikely to contain more than about 40 mg of tyramine. When MAO-A is inhibited, it may take as little as 10 mg of dietary tyramine to increase blood pressure (Figure 7-55). Because of the potential danger of a hypertensive crisis from a tyramine reaction in

Table 7-2 Hypertensive crisis

Defined by diastolic blood pressure > 120 mmHg
Potentially fatal reaction characterized by:

Occipital headache that may radiate frontally

Palpitation

Neck stiffness or soreness

Nausea

Vomiting

Sweating (sometimes with fever)

Dilated pupils, photophobia

Tachycardia or bradycardia, which can be associated with constricting chest pain

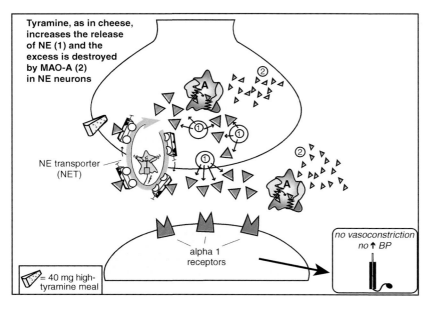

Tyramine, as in cheese, increases the release of NE (1) and the excess is destroyed by MAO-A (2) in NE neurons

NE transporter (NET)

alpha 1 receptors

no vasoconstriction no ↑ BP

= 40 mg high-tyramine meal

Figure 7-54. Tyramine increases norepinephrine release. Tyramine is an amine present in various foods, including cheese. Indicated in this figure is how a high-tyramine meal (40 mg, depicted here as cheese) acts to increase the release of norepinephrine (NE) (1). However, in normal circumstances the enzyme monoamine oxidase A (MAO-A) readily destroys the excess NE released by tyramine (2), and no harm is done (i.e., no vasoconstriction or elevation in blood pressure).

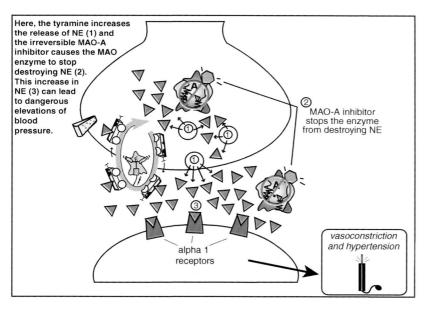

Here, the tyramine increases the release of NE (1) and the irreversible MAO-A inhibitor causes the MAO enzyme to stop destroying NE (2). This increase in NE (3) can lead to dangerous elevations of blood pressure.

MAO-A inhibitor stops the enzyme from destroying NE

alpha 1 receptors

vasoconstriction and hypertension

Figure 7-55. Inhibition of monoamine oxidase A (MAO-A) and tyramine. Here tyramine is releasing norepinephrine (NE) just as shown in Figure 7-54 (1). However, this time MAO-A is also being inhibited by an irreversible MAO-A inhibitor. This results in MAO-A stopping its destruction of NE (2). As indicated in Figure 7-51, such MAO-A inhibition in itself causes accumulation of NE. When MAO-A inhibition is taking place in the presence of tyramine, the combination can lead to a very large accumulation of NE (3). Such a great NE accumulation can lead to excessive stimulation of postsynaptic adrenergic receptors (3) and therefore dangerous vasoconstriction and elevation of blood pressure.

patients taking irreversible MAOIs, a certain mythology has grown up around how much tyramine is in various foods and therefore what dietary restrictions are necessary (Table 7-3). Since the tyramine reaction is sometimes called a "cheese reaction," there is a myth that all cheese must be restricted for a patient taking an MAOI. However, that is true only for aged cheeses, but not for most processed cheese or for most cheese utilized in most commercial chain pizzas. Also, it is not true that patients taking an MAOI must avoid all wine and beer. Canned and bottled beer are low in tyramine; generally only tap and nonpasteurized beers must be avoided, and many wines are actually quite low in tyramine. Of course, all prescribers should counsel patients taking the classic MAOIs about diet and keep up to date with the tyramine content of the foods their patients wish to eat (Table 7-3).

Table 7-3 Dietary guidelines for patients taking MAO inhibitors

The myth

If you're taking an MAOI, you can't eat cheese, drink wine or beer, or have many other foods that contain tyramine, or else you will develop hypertensive crisis.

The truth

There are a few things to avoid (which are easy to remember), but in practice diet is not really a problem …
… unless you plan to drink a gallon of blue cheese.

The Owner's Manual

Foods to avoid[a]	Foods allowed
Dried, aged, smoked, fermented, spoiled or improperly stored meat, poultry or fish	Fresh or processed meat, poultry and fish; properly stored pickled or smoked fish
Broad bean pods	All other vegetables
Aged cheeses	Processed cheese slices, cottage cheese, ricotta cheese, yogurt, cream cheese
Tap and unpasteurized beer	Canned or bottled beer and alcohol
Marmite	Brewer's and baker's yeast
Sauerkraut, kimchee	
Soy products/tofu	Peanuts
Banana peel	Bananas, avocados, raspberries
Tyramine-containing nutritional supplement	

[a] Not necessary for 6 mg transdermal or low-dose oral selegiline.

In fact, there are two MAOIs that do not require any dietary restrictions. Selegiline is a selective MAO-B inhibitor at low oral doses; administering low oral doses of selegiline does not have any dietary restrictions but also does not inhibit MAO-A in the brain and is therefore not an antidepressant. At high oral doses selegiline does inhibit MAO-A and therefore has antidepressant effects, but requires the need to restrict dietary tyramine. However, delivering selegiline through a transdermal patch allows inhibition of both MAO-A and MAO-B in the brain while largely bypassing inhibition of MAO-A in the gut (Figure 7-56). That is, transdermal delivery is like an intravenous infusion without the needle, delivering drug directly into the systemic circulation, hitting the brain in high doses, and avoiding a first pass through the liver (Figure 7-56). By the time the drug recirculates to the intestine and liver, it has much decreased levels and significantly inhibits only MAO-B in these tissues. This action is sufficiently robust and selective at low doses of transdermal selegiline, and thus no dietary tyramine restrictions are necessary. At high doses of transdermal selegiline, there is likely some MAO-A inhibition in the gut, and thus some dietary tyramine restrictions may be prudent.

Another mechanism to theoretically reduce risk of tyramine reactions is to use reversible inhibitors of MAO-A (RIMAs). Irreversible inhibition of MAO-A, as with the older MAOIs (Figure 7-54), prevents MAO-A from ever functioning again; enzyme activity returns only after new enzyme is synthesized. RIMAs, on the other hand, can be removed from the enzyme by competitive inhibition by MAO-A substrates (Figure 7-57). Thus, when tyramine releases norepinephrine, there is competition for MAO-A binding, and if norepinephrine levels are high enough, they can displace the RIMA from MAO-A and the enzyme activity is restored, allowing for the normal destruction of the extra norepinephrine and thereby reducing the risk of a tyramine reaction (Figure 7-57). However, the RIMA moclobemide still carries the dietary restriction warnings of irreversible MAOIs. A new

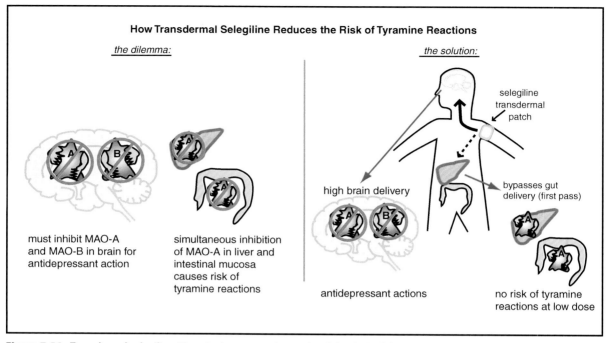

Figure 7-56. Transdermal selegiline. The selective monoamine oxidase B (MAO-B) inhibitor selegiline has antidepressant efficacy only when given at doses high enough also to inhibit monoamine oxidase A (MAO-A); yet when it is administered orally at these doses, it can also cause a tyramine reaction. How can selegiline inhibit both MAO-A and MAO-B in the brain, to have antidepressant effects, while inhibiting only MAO-B in the gut, so as to avoid a tyramine reaction? Transdermal administration of selegiline delivers the drug directly into the systemic circulation, hitting the brain in high doses and thus having antidepressant effects but avoiding a first pass through the liver and thus reducing risk of a tyramine reaction.

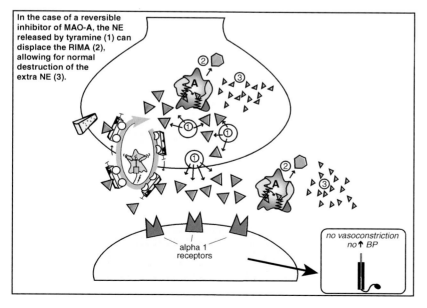

Figure 7-57. Reversible inhibition of monoamine oxidase A (MAO-A). Shown in this figure is the combination of an MAO-A inhibitor and tyramine. However, in this case the MAO-A inhibitor is of the reversible type (reversible inhibitor of MAO-A, or RIMA). The accumulation of norepinephrine (NE) released by tyramine (1) can displace the RIMA (2), allowing for normal destruction of the extra NE (3).

RIMA in late-stage clinical testing is TriRima (CX157) which will hopefully not require dietary restrictions.

Drug–drug interactions for MAOIs

While MAOIs are famous for their tyramine reactions, drug–drug interactions are potentially more important clinically. MAOI drug–drug interactions may not only be more common, but also some interactions can be dangerous or even lethal. Drug interactions with MAOIs are poorly understood by many practitioners. Since most candidates for MAOI treatment will require treatment with many concomitant drugs over time, including treatment for coughs and colds, and for pain, this can prevent psychopharmacologists from prescribing an MAOI if they do not know which drugs are safe to give and which ones must be avoided.

There are two general types of potentially dangerous drug interactions with MAOIs for a practitioner to understand and avoid: those that can raise blood pressure by sympathomimetic actions, and those that can cause a potentially fatal serotonin syndrome by serotonin reuptake inhibition.

MAOIs and sympathomimetics to avoid or administer with caution

When drugs that boost adrenergic stimulation by a mechanism other than MAO inhibition are added to an MAOI, potentially dangerous hypertensive reactions can occur. For example, decongestants stimulate postsynaptic α_1 receptors directly or indirectly (Figure 7-58A); this constricts nasal blood vessels, but does not typically elevate blood pressure at therapeutic doses when the decongestants are given by themselves. MAOIs elevate norepinephrine, but this alone does not typically elevate blood pressure either (Figure 7-58B). However, the direct α_1 stimulation of a decongestant combined with the elevation of norepinephrine that occurs when taking an MAOI may be sufficient to cause hypertension or even hypertensive crisis (Figure 7-58C). This is less likely with topical/intranasal administration and less likely in those not vulnerable to hypertension, but must be monitored in any patient taking a decongestant with an MAOI. Other agents that can increase noradrenergic activity include stimulants, some antidepressants, and others listed in Table 7-4. For patients with colds/upper respiratory infections, who are on MAOIs, it is probably best to use

antihistamines, which are safe with the exception of those that are also serotonin reuptake inhibitors (e.g., brompheniramine and chlorpheniramine) (Table 7-4). Cough medicines with expectorants or codeine are safe, but avoid dextromethorphan, a weak serotonin reuptake inhibitor.

MAOI interactions with anesthetics

Both general anesthesia and local anesthetics that contain epinephrine can cause changes in blood pressure (Table 7-4). Thus, for a patient taking an MAO inhibitor who needs to have a local anesthetic, one should choose an agent that does not contain vasoconstrictors (Table 7-5). For elective surgery, one should wash out the MAO inhibitor 10 days prior to the surgery (Table 7-5). For urgent surgery or elective surgery when the patient is still taking an MAO inhibitor, one can cautiously use a benzodiazepine, mivacurium, rapacuronium, morphine, or codeine (Table 7-5).

Avoid MAOIs with serotonergic agents

A potentially much more dangerous combination than that of adrenergic stimulants and MAOIs is the combination of agents that inhibit serotonin reuptake with those that inhibit MAO. Inhibition of the serotonin transporter (SERT) leads to therapeutic levels of increased synaptic availability of serotonin (Figure 7-59A), as does inhibition of MAO-A (Figure 7-59B). However, in combination, these two mechanisms can cause excessive stimulation of postsynaptic serotonin receptors, which has the potential to cause a fatal *serotonin syndrome* or *serotonin toxicity* (Figure 7-59C). The general clinical features of serotonin toxicity can range from migraines, myoclonus, agitation, and confusion on the mild end of the spectrum, to hyperthermia, seizures, coma, cardiovascular collapse, permanent hyperthermic brain damage, and even death at the severe end of the spectrum. Early diagnostic criteria for serotonin toxicity (syndrome) were developed by Sternbach based on examination of published case reports (Table 7-6). However, these criteria can lack both sensitivity and specificity. The apparent limitations of the Sternbach criteria for serotonin toxicity prompted Gilman's group in Australia to develop a set of diagnostic criteria called the Hunter Serotonin Toxicity Criteria based on retrospective analysis of more than 2200 patients who experienced overdose from a serotonergic drug (Table 7-7). Only five of the clinical features associated

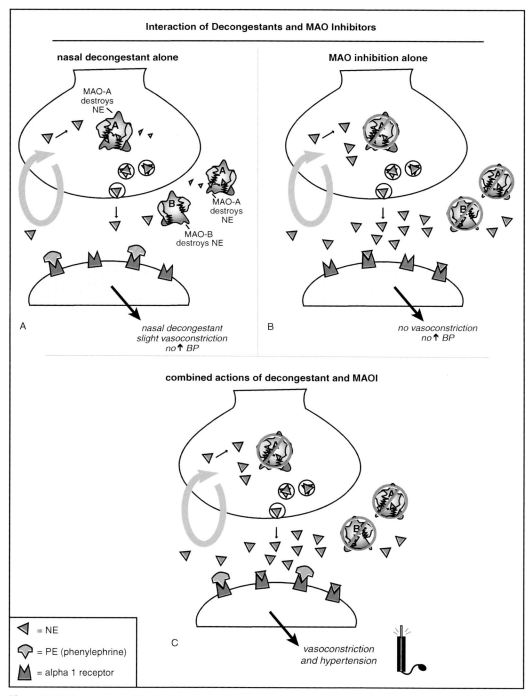

Figure 7-58. Interaction of decongestants and monoamine oxidase (MAO) inhibitors. Decongestants that stimulate postsynaptic α_1 receptors, such as phenylephrine, may interact with MAO inhibitors to increase risk of a tyramine reaction. Decongestants work by constricting nasal blood vessels, but they do not typically elevate blood pressure at the doses used (A). An MAO inhibitor given alone (and without the ingestion of tyramine) increases norepinephrine but does not usually cause vasoconstriction or hypertension (B). However, the noradrenergic actions of an MAO inhibitor combined with the direct α_1 stimulation of a decongestant may be sufficient to cause hypertension or even hypertensive crisis (C).

Table 7-4 Drugs that boost norepinephrine and thus should be used with caution with MAO inhibitors

The myth

If you're taking an MAOI, you can't take anything with norepinephrine reuptake inhibition, which means:

(1) You cannot have a local or a general anesthetic, so patients who need dental work, sutures, or surgery cannot take an MAOI.
(2) You can't take cold medications, such as decongestants, antihistamines, or cough medicines, so patients who get colds cannot take MAOIs.
(3) You can't take stimulants, so patients who need stimulants cannot take MAOIs.

The truth

Be careful using local anesthetics that contain epinephrine, and using general anesthesia, as these can cause blood pressure changes.

Sympathomimetic decongestants and stimulants should be used with caution while monitoring blood pressure in patients for whom the benefits are greater than the risks, and should be avoided only in high-risk/low-benefit populations.

The Owner's Manual: use with caution*

Decongestants	Stimulants	Antidepressants with norepineprhine reuptake inhibition	Other
Phenylephrine	Amphetamine	Most tricyclics	Phentermine
Pseudoephedrine	Methylphenidate	NRIs	Local anesthetics containing vasoconstrictors
	Modafinil	SNRIs	Tramadol, tapentadol
	Armodafinil	NDRIs	Cocaine, methamphetamine

* Some of these drugs may also have serotonergic properties that require contraindication with MAOIs.
NDRI, norepinephrine–dopamine reuptake inhibitor; NRI, norepinephrine reuptake inhibitor; SNRI, serotonin–norepinephrine reuptake inhibitor.

Table 7-5 The Owner's Manual: use of anesthetics

Local anesthetic	Elective surgery	Urgent or elective surgery when patient is still taking an MAO inhibitor
Choose an agent that does not contain vasoconstrictors	Wash out the MAO inhibitor 10 days prior to surgery	Cautiously use a benzodiazepine, mivacurium, rapacuronium, morphine, or codeine

Table 7-6 Serotonin toxicity: Sternbach criteria

Recent addition of or increase in a known serotonergic agent

Absence of other possible etiologies (infection, substance abuse, withdrawal, etc.)

No recent addition or increase of a neuroleptic agent

At least three of the following:

- Agitation
- Myoclonus
- Hyperreflexia
- Diaphoresis
- Shivering
- Tremor
- Diarrhea
- Ataxia/incoordination
- Fever

with serotonin toxicity were needed to make an accurate diagnosis: clonus, agitation, diaphoresis, tremor, and hyperreflexia. In addition, hypertonicity and hyperpyrexia were present in all life-threatening cases of serotonin toxicity. They also developed decision rules for diagnosis, based on the presence or absence of the seven clinical features (Table 7-7).

Drugs to avoid in combination with MAOIs in order to prevent serotonin toxicity are listed in Table 7-8. One can essentially never combine agents that have potent serotonin reuptake inhibition with

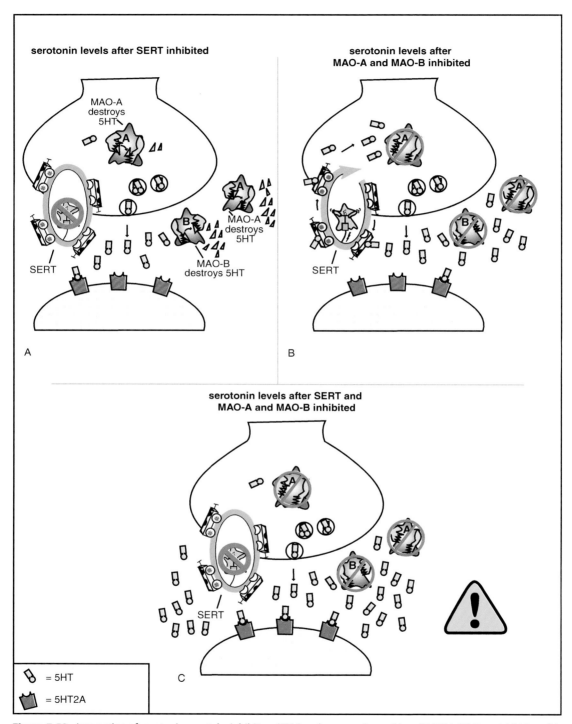

Figure 7-59. Interaction of serotonin reuptake inhibitors (SRIs) and monoamine oxidase (MAO) inhibitors. Inhibition of the serotonin transporter (SERT) leads to increased synaptic availability of serotonin (A). Similarly, inhibition of MAO leads to increased serotonin levels (B). These two mechanisms in combination can cause excessive stimulation of postsynaptic serotonin receptors, which may lead to hyperthermia, seizures, coma, cardiovascular collapse, or even death (C).

Table 7-7 Serotonin toxicity: Hunter criteria

Clinical features	Decision rules: in the presence of a serotonergic agent
Clonus	IF (spontaneous clonus = yes) THEN serotonin toxicity = YES
Agitation	OR ELSE IF (inducible clonus = yes) AND (agitation = yes) OR (diaphoresis = yes) THEN serotonin toxicity = YES
Diaphoresis	OR ELSE IF (ocular clonus = yes) AND (agitation = yes) OR (diaphoresis = yes) THEN serotonin toxicity = YES
Tremor	OR ELSE IF (tremor = yes) AND (hyperreflexia = yes) THEN serotonin toxicity = YES
Hyperreflexia	OR ELSE IF (hypertonic = yes) AND (temperature >38 °C) AND (ocular clonus = yes) OR (inducible clonus = yes) THEN serotonin toxicity = YES
Hypertonicity	OR ELSE serotonin toxicity = NO
Hyperpyrexia	

agents given in doses that cause substantial MAO inhibition. This includes any selective serotonin reuptake inhibitor (SSRI), any serotonin–norepinephrine reuptake inhibitor (SNRI), and the tricyclic antidepressant clomipramine. Opioids that block serotonin reuptake, especially meperidine but also tramadol, and dextromethorphan, must also be avoided when an MAO inhibitor is given (Table 7-8). Several drugs of abuse also block serotonin reuptake: thus, diligent questioning about drug use/abuse is necessary when considering prescribing an MAO inhibitor (Table 7-8). Although it is commonly believed that serotonin 1A partial agonism or the proserotonergic actions of lithium could also contribute to serotonin syndrome in combination with an MAOI, these mechanisms are not actually contraindications, and such medications can be administered with caution by experts in combination with an MAOI.

MAOI interactions with TCAs

MAOIs are formally contraindicated in the prescribing information for patients taking antidepressants that are norepinephrine reuptake inhibitors, such as most tricyclic antidepressants. This is because the sudden addition of noradrenergic reuptake blockade

Table 7-8 Drugs to avoid in combination with an MAO inhibitor due to the risk of serotonin syndrome/toxicity

The myth

You can't take any medications that block serotonin reuptake, which means you can't take any psychotropic medications. Since all patients who are candidates for an MAOI need concomitant medications, no one can take an MAOI.

Besides, you cannot get there from here because in order to start an MAOI, you have to disrupt everything, stopping all other meds for 2 weeks after taper. And, if you have to stop an MAOI to go back to a psychotropic medication, you have to go without all meds for another 2 weeks. This is an unacceptable risk and a hassle.

The truth

You must avoid only agents that block serotonin reuptake. There are many options for not only bridging between serotonin reuptake inhibitors and MAOIs, but also augmenting MAOIs.

The Owner's Manual: do not use

Antidepressants	Drugs of abuse	Opioids	Other
SSRIs	MDMA (ecstasy)	Meperidine	Non-subcutaneous sumatriptan
SNRIs	Cocaine	Tramadol	Chlorpheniramine
Clomipramine	Methamphetamine	Methadone	Brompheniramine
St. John's wort	High-dose or injected amphetamine	Fentanyl	Procarbazine?
			Dextromethorphan

MDMA, 3,4-methylenedioxymethamphetamine; SNRI, serotonin–norepinephrine reuptake inhibitor; SSRI, selective serotonin reuptake inhibitor.

in someone on an MAOI may result in a hypertensive reaction. However, with the exception of clomipramine, a potent serotonin reuptake inhibitor, other tricyclic antidepressants can be combined with MAOIs with caution for severely treatment-resistant patients by experts doing careful monitoring (Table 7-9). If this option is selected, one should start the MAO inhibitor at the same time as the tricyclic antidepressant (both at low doses) after an appropriate drug washout; then, one should alternately increase the doses of these agents every few days to a week as tolerated. The MAOI should not be started first.

Cyclobenzaprine, carbamazepine, and oxcarbazepine are structurally related to tricyclic antidepressants, and therefore some individuals believe they cannot be used with MAOIs; however, these agents do not block serotonin or norepinephrine reuptake and thus can be used with caution (Table 7-9).

MAOI interactions with opioids

Contrary to popular opinion, there is no dangerous pharmacological interaction between MAOIs and opioid mechanisms; instead, the reason why some opioids must be avoided is that certain agents (especially meperidine; possibly methadone and tramadol) have concomitant serotonin reuptake inhibition, while another (tapentadol) has norepinephrine reuptake inhibition (Table 7-10). Analgesics, including opioids, which are safe to administer with an MAOI are those lacking serotonin reuptake inhibiting properties, such as aspirin, acetaminophen, nonsteroidal anti-inflammatory drugs (NSAIDs), codeine, hydrocodone, and some others (Table 7-10).

Switching to and from MAOIs, and bridging medications to use during the switches

Because of the risk of serotonin toxicity, complete washout of a serotonergic drug is necessary before starting an MAO inhibitor (Figure 7-60). One must wait at least 5 half-lives after discontinuing the serotonergic drug before starting the MAO inhibitor. For most drugs, this means waiting 5–7 days; a notable exception is fluoxetine, for which one must wait 5 weeks because of

Table 7-9 The Owner's Manual: using tricyclic antidepressants with MAO inhibitors

Contraindicated	Use with caution
Clomipramine	Other tricyclic antidepressants
	Cyclobenzaprine
	Carbamazepine
	Oxcarbazepine

Table 7-10 Combining MAO inhibitors and pain medications

The myth

If you're taking an MAOI, you can't take painkillers because they will kill you, so patients who have sprained ankles, sore muscles, dental extractions, or surgeries cannot take MAOIs, as they must avoid all opioid and non-opioid painkillers.

The truth

There are a few things to avoid (which are easy to remember), and in practice, this is not really a problem.

The Owner's Manual

Use with MAOIs

Should be fine	Should be cautious	May sometimes be done by experts	Is not recommended	Is strictly prohibited
Acetaminophen	Buprenorphine	Hydromorphone	Fentanyl	Meperidine
Aspirin	Butorphanol	Morphine	Methadone	
NSAIDs	Codeine	Oxycodone	Tapentadol	
	Hydrocodone	Oxymorphone	Tramadol	
	Nalbuphine			
	Pentazocine			

its long half-life and the long half-life of its active metabolite norfluoxetine.

When switching in the other direction, namely from an MAOI to a serotonin reuptake inhibitor, one must wait at least 14 days following the discontinuation of the MAO inhibitor before starting the serotonergic drug, to allow regeneration of sufficient MAO enzyme (Figure 7-61).

Because there is a required gap in antidepressant treatment when switching to or from an MAO inhibitor, clinicians may be concerned about managing symptoms during that time period. There are many medication options, depending on the individual patient's situation. These include benzodiazepines, Z-drug sedative hypnotics (e.g., zolpidem, eszopiclone, zaleplon), trazodone, lamotrigine, valproate, several other anticonvulsants, stimulants, and atypical antipsychotics (Table 7-11). Specifically, although trazodone does have serotonin reuptake inhibition at

Table 7-11 The Owner's Manual: how to bridge

Use these drugs with caution and careful monitoring while waiting to start an MAOI or when discontinuing an MAOI

Benzodiazepines

Z-drug hypnotics

Trazodone

Lamotrigine

Valproate

Gabapentin, pregabalin, topiramate, carbamazepine, oxcarbazepine

Stimulants

Atypical antipsychotics

Switching From a Serotonergic Drug to an MAOI

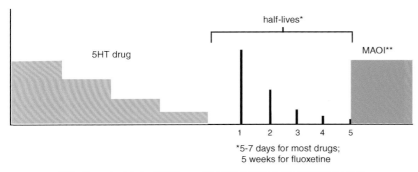

Figure 7-60. **Switching from a serotonergic drug to an MAOI.** Because of the risk of serotonin toxicity, complete washout of a serotonergic drug is necessary before starting an MAOI. One must wait at least 5 half-lives after discontinuing the serotonergic drug before starting the MAOI. For most drugs, this means waiting 5–7 days; a notable exception is fluoxetine, for which one must wait 5 weeks due to its long half-life.

Switching From an MAOI to a Serotonergic Drug

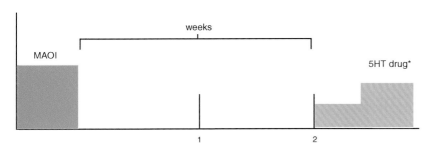

Figure 7-61. **Switching from an MAOI to a serotonergic drug.** If one is switching from an MAOI to a serotonin reuptake inhibitor, one must wait at least 14 days following the discontinuation of the MAOI before starting the serotonergic drug.

antidepressant doses (i.e., 150 mg or higher), this property is not clinically relevant at the low doses used for insomnia while bridging an MAO inhibitor. The atypical antipsychotic ziprasidone also has serotonin reuptake inhibition, and is probably best avoided.

The bottom line for MAOIs

MAOIs should not be discounted as valuable treatment options for treatment-resistant depression and some treatment-resistant anxiety disorders such as panic disorder and social anxiety disorder. Although use of an MAOI does require a watchful eye over dietary intake, the restrictions are not as widespread as many believe. Likewise, although drug interactions can be serious and concomitant medication use must be stringently overseen, there are some mistaken beliefs regarding the extent of the medication mechanisms that must be avoided. Armed with knowledge of MAOI therapeutic, dietary, and drug-interaction mechanisms, clinicians may be able to revive these agents as therapeutic tools in the fight against treatment-resistant depression and anxiety.

Classic antidepressants: tricyclic antidepressants

The tricyclic antidepressants (TCAs) (Table 7-12; Figure 7-62) were so named because their chemical structure contains three rings. The TCAs were

Table 7-12 Some tricyclic antidepressants still in use

Generic name	Trade name
Clomipramine	Anafranil
Imipramine	Tofranil
Amitriptyline	Elavil; Endep; Tryprizol; Loroxyl
Nortriptyline	Pamelor; Endep; Aventyl
Protriptyline	Vivactil
Maprotiline	Ludiomil
Amoxapine	Asendin
Doxepin	Sinequan; Adapin
Desipramine	Norpramin; Pertofran
Trimipramine	Surmontil
Dothiepin	Prothiaden
Lofepramine	Deprimyl; Gamanil
Tianeptine	Coaxil; Stablon

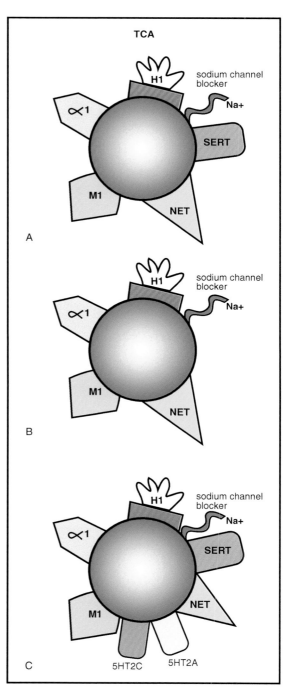

Figure 7-62. Icons of tricyclic antidepressants. All tricyclic antidepressants block reuptake of norepinephrine and are antagonists at H_1-histaminic, α_1-adrenergic, and muscarinic cholinergic receptors; they also block voltage-sensitive sodium channels (A, B, and C). Some tricyclic antidepressants are also potent inhibitors of the serotonin reuptake pump (A), and some may additionally be antagonists at serotonin 2A and 2C receptors (C).

synthesized about the same time as other three-ringed molecules which were shown to be effective tranquilizers for schizophrenia (i.e., the early antipsychotic neuroleptic drugs such as chlorpromazine) but were a disappointment when tested as antipsychotics. However, during testing for schizophrenia, they were discovered to be antidepressants. Long after their antidepressant properties were observed, the tricyclic antidepressants were discovered to block the reuptake pumps for norepinephrine (i.e., NET), or for both norepinephrine and serotonin (i.e., SERT) (Figures 7-62, 7-63, 7-64). Some tricyclics have equal or greater potency for SERT inhibition

(e.g., clomipramine: Figure 7-62A); others are more selective for NET inhibition (e.g., desipramine, maprotiline, nortriptyline, protriptyline: Figure 7-62B). Most, however, block both serotonin and norepinephrine reuptake to some extent. In addition, some tricyclic antidepressants have antagonist actions at $5HT_{2A}$ and $5HT_{2C}$ receptors which could contribute to their therapeutic profile (Figures 7-62C, 7-65, 7-66).

The major limitation to the tricyclic antidepressants has never been their efficacy: these are quite effective agents. The problem with drugs in this class is the fact that all of them share at least four other

SRI Inserted

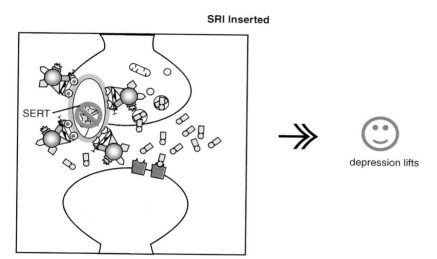

depression lifts

Figure 7-63. Therapeutic actions of tricyclic antidepressants (TCAs), part 1. In this figure, the TCA is shown with its serotonin reuptake inhibitor (SRI) portion inserted into the serotonin transporter (SERT), blocking it and causing an antidepressant effect.

NRI Inserted

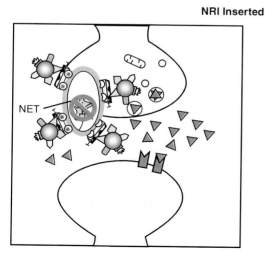

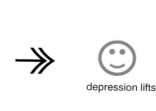

depression lifts

Figure 7-64. Therapeutic actions of tricyclic antidepressants (TCAs), part 2. In this figure, the TCA is shown with its norepinephrine reuptake inhibitor (NRI) portion inserted into the norepinephrine transporter (NET), blocking it and causing an antidepressant effect. Thus both the serotonin reuptake portion (Figure 7-63) and the norepinephrine reuptake portion of the TCA act pharmacologically to cause an antidepressant effect.

5HT2A Inserted

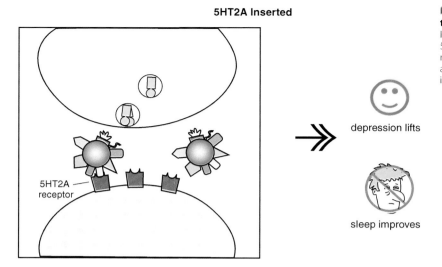

Figure 7-65. Therapeutic actions of tricyclic antidepressants (TCAs), part 3. In this figure, the TCA is shown with its 5HT$_{2A}$ portion inserted into the 5HT$_{2A}$ receptor, blocking it and causing an antidepressant effect as well as potentially improving sleep.

depression lifts

sleep improves

5HT2C Inserted

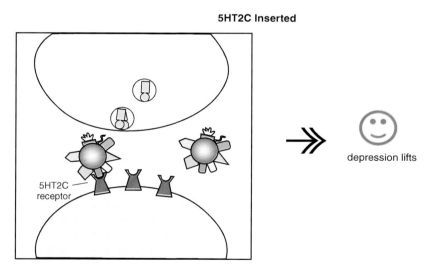

Figure 7-66. Therapeutic actions of tricyclic antidepressants (TCAs), part 4. In this figure, the TCA is shown with its 5HT$_{2C}$ portion inserted into the 5HT$_{2C}$ receptor, blocking it and causing an antidepressant effect.

depression lifts

unwanted pharmacologic actions, shown in Figure 7-62: namely, blockade of muscarinic cholinergic receptors, H$_1$-histaminic receptors, α$_1$-adrenergic receptors, and voltage-sensitive sodium channels (Figures 7-67 through 7-70).

Blockade of H$_1$-histaminic receptors, also called antihistaminic action, causes sedation and may cause weight gain (Figure 7-67). Blockade of M$_1$-muscarinic cholinergic receptors, also known as anticholinergic actions, causes dry mouth, blurred vision, urinary retention, and constipation (Figure

7-68). Blockade of α$_1$-adrenergic receptors causes orthostatic hypotension and dizziness (Figure 7-69). Tricyclic antidepressants also weakly block voltage-sensitive sodium channels (VSSCs) in heart and brain, and in overdose this action is thought to be the cause of coma and seizures due to central nervous system actions, and cardiac arrhythmias and cardiac arrest and death due to peripheral cardiac actions (Figure 7-70).

Tricyclic antidepressants are not merely antidepressants, since one of them (clomipramine)

H1 Inserted

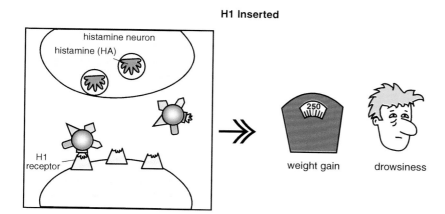

weight gain   drowsiness

Figure 7-67. Side effects of tricyclic antidepressants (TCAs), part 1. In this figure, the TCA is shown with its antihistamine (H₁) portion inserted into histamine receptors, causing the side effects of weight gain and drowsiness.

M1 Inserted

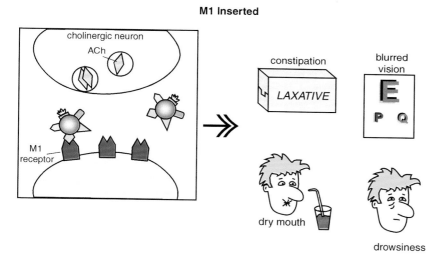

constipation   blurred vision

LAXATIVE

dry mouth   drowsiness

Figure 7-68. Side effects of tricyclic antidepressants (TCAs), part 2. In this figure, the TCA is shown with its anticholinergic/antimuscarinic (M₁) portion inserted into acetylcholine receptors, causing the side effects of constipation, blurred vision, dry mouth, and drowsiness.

∝ 1 Inserted

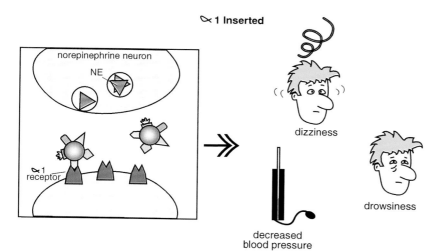

dizziness

decreased blood pressure   drowsiness

Figure 7-69. Side effects of tricyclic antidepressants (TCAs), part 3. In this figure, the TCA is shown with its α-adrenergic antagonist portion inserted into α₁-adrenergic receptors, causing the side effects of dizziness, drowsiness, and decreased blood pressure.

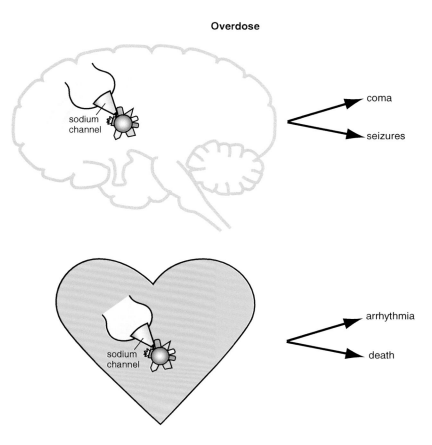

Overdose

Figure 7-70. Side effects of tricyclic antidepressants (TCAs), part 4. In this figure, the TCA is shown with its sodium channel blocker portion blocking voltage-sensitive sodium channels in the brain (top) and heart (bottom). In overdose, this action can lead to coma, seizures, arrhythmia, and even death.

has anti-obsessive–compulsive disorder effects and many of them have anti-panic effects at antidepressant doses and efficacy for neuropathic and low back pain at low doses. Because of their side effects and potential for death in overdose, tricyclic antidepressants have fallen into second-line use for depression.

Augmenting antidepressants

An increasing number of agents, devices, and procedures are now utilized alone or in combination with standard antidepressants to augment antidepressant efficacy in patients who do not attain full remission. The use of atypical antipsychotics as augmenting agents to antidepressants, and the hypothetical mechanism of their action in depression, is discussed extensively in Chapter 5. Above we have mentioned the combination of the 5HT$_{1A}$ partial agonist buspirone with SSRIs in the section covering vilazodone.

Lithium is discussed in Chapter 8 on mood stabilizers. Here, we mention various natural products, hormones, neurostimulation therapies, and psychotherapies as alternatives or as augmentation to antidepressants.

L-5-Methyltetrahydrofolate (L-methylfolate): monoamine modulator

L-Methylfolate, synthesized in the body from folate or dihydrofolate in the diet (Figure 7-71) or available as a medical food by prescription and called Deplin in the US, is an important regulator of a critical cofactor for monoamine neurotransmitter synthesis, namely tetrahydrobiopterin or BH4 (Figure 7-72). The monoamine synthetic enzymes that require BH4 as a cofactor are both tryptophan hydroxylase, the rate-limiting enzyme for serotonin synthesis, and tyrosine hydroxylase, the rate-limiting enzyme not only for dopamine synthesis but also for norepinephrine

Formation of L-methylfolate from Folic Acid (F)

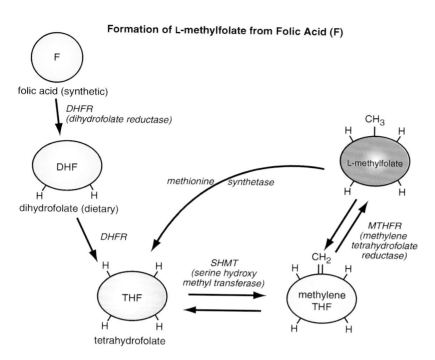

Figure 7-71. Formation of L-methylfolate from folic acid (F). L-Methylfolate is a monoamine modulator naturally synthesized from the vitamin folate for use within the central nervous system. Folic acid (synthetic) is converted to dihydrofolate (DHF) by the enzyme dihydrofolate reductase (DHFR), and DHF, in turn, is converted to tetrahydrofolate (THF), again by DHFR. Serine hydroxymethyl-transferase (SHMT) then converts THF to methylene THF. Finally, methylene THF is converted by methylene tetrahydrofolate reductase (MTHFR) to L-methylfolate.

BH4 Cofactor for Monoamine Neurotransmitter Synthesis

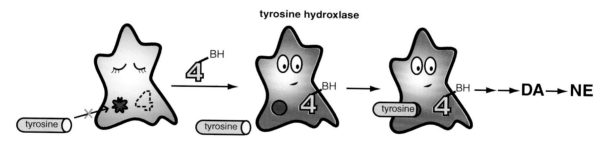

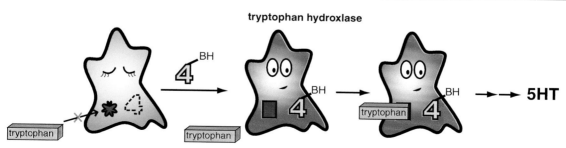

Figure 7-72. Tetrahydrobiopterin (BH4) cofactor for monoamine neurotransmitter synthesis. BH4 is a critical enzyme cofactor for tyrosine hydroxylase, the rate-limiting enzyme for dopamine and norepinephrine synthesis, and tryptophan hydroxylase, the rate-limiting enzyme for serotonin. Because L-methylfolate regulates BH4 production, it therefore plays an indirect role in regulating monoamine synthesis and concentrations.

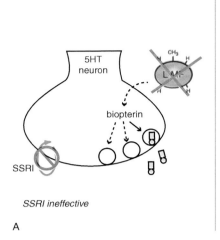

SSRI ineffective

A

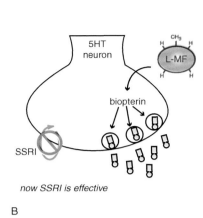

now SSRI is effective

B

Figure 7-73. **Folate deficiency and monoamines.** (A) Because L-methylfolate (L-MF) indirectly regulates monoamine neurotransmitter synthesis, deficiency of folate, from which it is derived, can lead to reduced monoamine levels and thus to symptoms of depression. Reduced synthesis of monoamines may mean that, even in the presence of a selective serotonin reuptake inhibitor (SSRI), serotonin levels may remain low. In fact, studies show that low levels of folate or L-MF may be linked to depression in some patients. (B) Administration of L-MF, folate, or folinic acid in conjunction with an antidepressant may boost the therapeutic effects of antidepressant monotherapy. High doses of oral L-MF may be the most efficient of these for boosting BH4 production in the central nervous system and thus enhancing brain monoamine neurotransmitter levels.

synthesis (Figure 7-72). Low amounts of L-methylfolate from genetic and/or environmental/dietary causes could theoretically lead to low synthesis of monoamines (Figures 7-73 and 7-74) and contribute to depression or to the resistance of some patients to treatment with antidepressants. That is, antidepressants such as SSRIs/SNRIs and others rely upon the continued synthesis of monoamines in order to work (Figure 7-73A). If there are no monoamines released, reuptake blockade is ineffective (Figure 7-73A). However, repletion of monoamine synthesis by L-methylfolate would theoretically make such patients responsive to antidepressants (Figure 7-73B).

A second mechanism involving L-methylfolate theoretically influences monoamine levels. That is, methylation of genes silences them, as discussed in Chapter 1 and illustrated in Figure 1-30. L-Methylfolate provides the methyl group for this silencing, so if L-methylfolate is low, potentially silencing of various genes could also be low. Specifically, if the silencing of the gene for the enzyme COMT (catechol-O-methyl-transferase) is low, more copies of this enzyme are made and enzyme activity goes up, causing dopamine levels to go down particularly in prefrontal cortex, potentially compromising information processing and causing symptoms such as cognitive dysfunction (Figure 7-74A). Hypothetically, silencing of COMT synthesis by L-methylfolate could result in higher dopamine levels in prefrontal cortex and improve symptoms linked to dopamine deficiency, such as cognitive deficits (Figure 7-74B).

What could cause problems in L-methylfolate availability that might lead to inefficient functioning of monoamine neurotransmitters? Some patients have dietary deficiencies severe enough to result in low levels of folate (or reciprocally high levels of homocysteine). In others, the deficiency in L-methylfolate may be more functional than manifest as low blood levels, and linked instead to genetic variants in folate metabolism. Several genetic variants exist in enzymes that regulate L-methylfolate levels:

- Methylene tetrahydrofolate reductase: MTHFR C677T; MTHFR A1298C
- Methionine synthase: MTR A2756G
- Methionine synthase reductase: MTRR A66G

Inheriting variants of these enzymes that lead to less availability of L-methylfolate could potentially compromise monoamine levels by impacting their synthesis and metabolism (Figures 7-73 and 7-74). This in turn could hypothetically contribute either to the cause of depression or some symptoms of depression, or be linked to treatment resistance. Evidence for this is only beginning to accumulate, including who might be the best candidates with depression for treatment with L-methylfolate (in contrast to folate) that would bypass these genetic variants. One hint comes from studies of MTHFR and COMT in schizophrenia (discussed in Chapter 4) and suggests that effects of some gene variants on the efficiency of information processing might be greater if variants in two or more particular genes are inherited together (see Figure 4-44).

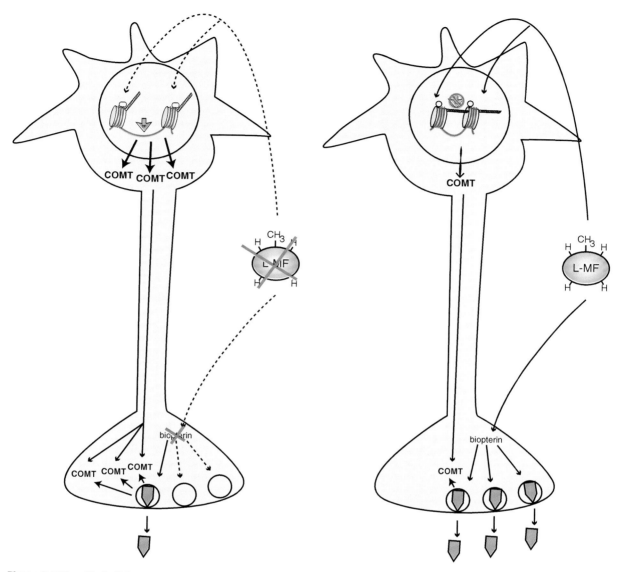

Figure 7-74A. L-Methylfolate and COMT, part 1. L-Methylfolate (L-MF) assists in the formation of tetrahydrobiopterin (biopterin), which is a critical cofactor for the synthesis of monoamines including dopamine. In addition, L-methylfolate could hypothetically lead to methylation of the promoter for the gene of the enzyme COMT (catechol-*O*-methyl-transferase), which inactivates dopamine and norepinephrine. This methylation silences the gene and decreases the synthesis of COMT enzyme, which reduces the metabolism of dopamine and norepinephrine. When L-methylfolate is deficient, biopterin formation is reduced and thus it is not sufficiently present to activate the enzyme that synthesizes dopamine, and dopamine levels are reduced. Furthermore, in the absence of L-methylfolate, methylation of the gene for COMT is reduced, leading to activation of this gene and thus increasing COMT synthesis. This in turn increases dopamine metabolism, further reducing dopamine levels.

Figure 7-74B. L-Methylfolate and COMT, part 2. When L-methylfolate (L-MF) is present, it can assist in the formation of tetrahydrobiopterin (biopterin), which is a critical cofactor for the synthesis of dopamine: thus dopamine levels will increase. In addition, L-methylfolate can hypothetically increase methylation of the promoter for the gene of the enzyme COMT (catechol-*O*-methyl-transferase), which inactivates dopamine. This methylation silences the COMT gene and thus decreases the synthesis of COMT, which reduces the metabolism of dopamine, increasing its levels.

The effects of two or more risk genes working together to increase the risk of an illness such as depression is called *epistasis*. There is some evidence that the T variant of MTHFR "conspires" with the Val variant of COMT to decrease the efficiency of information processing in the dorsolateral prefrontal cortex (DLPFC) during a cognitive load in schizophrenia ("having T with Val" in Chapter 4 and in Figure 4-44). This observation suggests the possibility that the same genetic interaction may be at play in some patients with depression, or treatment-resistant depression, or even depression with cognitive symptoms, and it is being explored as a potential genetic marker for who might be the best candidates for L-methylfolate treatment in depression.

S-adenosyl-methionine (SAMe)

L-Methylfolate is converted into methionine and finally into SAMe, which is the direct methyl donor for methylation reactions. If L-methylfolate is deficient, so might be SAMe, and it may be possible to administer methionine or SAMe to such patients as well as L-methylfolate. However, administering methionine or SAMe can cause build-up of the unwanted metabolite homocysteine that could theoretically interfere with epigenetic mechanisms, and can also eventually deplete precursors to SAMe. Nevertheless, high doses of SAMe may be effective in augmenting antidepressants in patients with major depression.

Thyroid

Thyroid hormones act by binding to nuclear ligand receptors to form a nuclear ligand-activated transcription factor. Abnormalities in thyroid hormone levels have long been associated with depression, and various forms and doses of thyroid hormones have long been utilized as augmenting agents to antidepressants, either to boost their efficacy in patients with inadequate response or to speed up their onset of action. Thyroid hormones have many complex cellular actions, including actions that may boost monoamine neurotransmitters as downstream consequences of thyroid's known abilities to regulate neuronal organization, arborization, and synapse formation, and this may account for how thyroid hormones enhance antidepressant action in some patients.

Brain stimulation: creating a perfect storm in brain circuits of depressed patients

Electroconvulsive therapy

Electroconvulsive therapy (ECT) is the classic therapeutic form of brain stimulation for depression. ECT is a highly effective treatment for depression whose mechanism of action remains a quandary. Failure to respond to a variety of antidepressants, singly or in combination, is a key factor for considering ECT, although it may also be utilized in urgent and severely disabling high-risk circumstances such as psychotic, suicidal, or postpartum depressions. ECT is the only therapeutic agent for the treatment of depression, with the possible exception of the experimental agents ketamine, scopolamine, and sleep deprivation, that is rapid in antidepressant onset, with therapeutic actions that can start after even a single treatment, and typically within a few days. The mechanism is unknown, but thought to be related to the probable mobilization of neurotransmitters caused by the seizure. Memory loss and social stigma are the primary problems associated with ECT and limit its use. There are striking regional and national differences across the world in the frequency of ECT use and in ECT techniques.

Transcranial magnetic stimulation

Transcranial magnetic stimulation (TMS) is another brain stimulation treatment approved for depression. It uses a rapidly alternating current passing through a small coil placed over the scalp that generates a magnetic field which in turn induces an electric current in the underlying areas of the brain. This electrical current depolarizes the affected cortical neurons, thereby causing nerve impulse flow out of the underlying brain areas (Figure 7-75). During the treatment the patient is awake and reclines comfortably in a chair while the magnetic coil is placed snugly against the scalp. There are few if any side effects except headache.

The TMS apparatus is localized in order to create an electrical impulse over the dorsolateral prefrontal cortex (DLPFC). Presumably, daily stimulation of this brain area for up to an hour over several weeks causes activation of various brain circuits that leads to an antidepressant effect (Figure 7-75). If this activates a brain circuit beginning in DLPFC, and connecting to other brain areas such as ventromedial prefrontal cortex (VMPFC) and amygdala, with connections to the brainstem centers of the monoamine neurotransmitter system, the net result would be monoamine

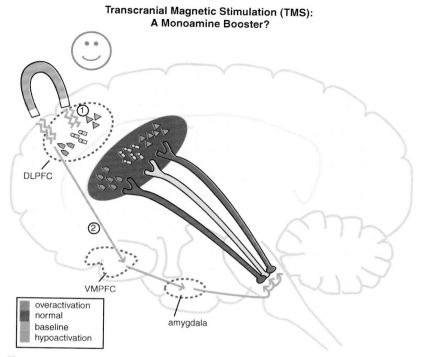

Figure 7-75. Transcranial magnetic stimulation. Transcranial magnetic stimulation is a treatment in which a rapidly alternating current passes through a small coil placed over the scalp. This generates a magnetic field that induces an electrical current in the underlying areas of the brain (dorsolateral prefrontal cortex, DLPFC). The affected neurons then signal other areas of the brain. Presumably, stimulation of brain regions in which there is monoamine deficiency would lead to a boost in monoamine activity and thus alleviation of depressive symptoms.

modulation, especially for patients inadequately responsive to treatment with antidepressants (Figure 7-75, arrow 2). In this way, TMS would act through a mechanism unlike the known chemical antidepressants. However, TMS also releases neurotransmitters locally, in the area of the magnet, depolarizing them and releasing neurotransmitters from their axon terminals in the DLPFC (Figure 7-75, arrow 1). This is a second mechanism unlike chemical antidepressants, and may explain why TMS can be effective in patients who do not respond to chemical antidepressants. Finally, since all the effects of TMS are in the brain, there are no peripheral side effects such as nausea, weight gain, blood pressure changes, or sexual dysfunction. Lack of peripheral side effects plus the ability to help patients who do not respond to chemical antidepressants seem to be the particular advantages of TMS treatment of depression.

Deep brain stimulation

Deep brain stimulation (DBS) is an experimental treatment for the most severe forms of depression (Figure 7-76). Deep brain stimulation of neurons in some brain areas has proven effective for treatment of motor complications in Parkinson's disease and is now under study for treatment-resistant depression. The stimulation device is a battery-powered pulse generator implanted in the chest wall like a pacemaker. One or two leads are tunneled under the scalp and then into the brain, guided by neuroimaging and brain stimulation recording during the implantation procedure to facilitate the exact placement of the lead in the targeted brain area. The tip of each lead is composed of several contact areas that usually spread sequentially to cover additional parts of the intended anatomic target. The pulse generator delivers brief repeated pulses of current, which is adjusted based on individual tissue impedence.

The most common side effects are from the procedure itself. There is ongoing debate on where to place the stimulating electrodes for the treatment of depression, and how such stimulation might work to treat depression in patients inadequately responsive to antidepressants. Currently, one proposed location for electrodes in the treatment of depression with deep

Deep Brain Stimulation (DBS): A Monoamine Booster?

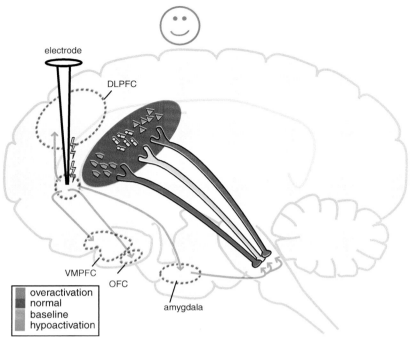

Figure 7-76. Deep brain stimulation. Deep brain stimulation involves a battery-powered pulse generator implanted in the chest wall. One or two leads are tunneled directly into the brain. The device then sends brief repeated pulses to the brain, which may have the result of boosting monoamine activity and thus alleviating depressive symptoms.

brain stimulation is in the subgenual area of the anterior cingulate cortex, part of the ventromedial prefrontal cortex (VMPFC: Figure 7-76). This brain area has important connections to other areas of prefrontal cortex, including other areas of ventromedial prefrontal cortex, orbitofrontal cortex (OFC), and dorsolateral prefrontal cortex, as well as amygdala (Figure 7-76). It is feasible that electrical stimulation of this brain area results in activation of circuits that lead back to brainstem monoamine centers, to act as a monoamine modulator in such patients. Reports of this treatment approach are encouraging.

Psychotherapy as an epigenetic "drug"

Psychotherapy has traditionally competed with psychopharmacology. As drugs have become the more dominant treatment, the pharmacological approach has been increasingly criticized as limited in scope, lacking in robust outcomes, and too heavily influenced by the pharmaceutical industry. However, drugs and psychotherapy may have a common neurobiological link since both can change brain circuits. It is not surprising, therefore, that both psychotherapy

and psychopharmacology can be clinically effective for treating psychiatric disorders, or indeed that combining them can be therapeutically synergistic. Psychotherapy, like many other forms of learning, can hypothetically induce epigenetic changes in brain circuits that can enhance the efficiency of information processing in malfunctioning neurons to improve symptoms in psychiatric disorders, just like drugs.

Psychotherapies can thus be conceptualized as epigenetic "drugs," or at least as therapeutic agents that act epigenetically in a manner similar or complementary to drugs. Inefficient information processing in specific circuits correlates with specific psychiatric symptoms. Not only can genes and psychotropic drugs modify various neurotransmitter systems to alter the activity of these circuits and thus create or alleviate psychiatric symptoms by changing the efficiency of information processing in these circuits, but so can environmental experiences such as stress (see Figures 6-40 through 6-43), learning, and possibly even psychotherapy. Drugs can change gene expression in brain circuits as a downstream consequence of their immediate molecular properties, but so can the environment, hypothetically including psychotherapy. That is, both good and bad experiences can drive the production of epigenetic changes in gene expression, and indeed epigenetic changes in gene transcription seem to underlie long-term memories, good and bad. Bad memories of childhood trauma may trigger psychiatric disorders by causing unfavorable changes in brain circuits; good memories formed during psychotherapy may favorably alter the same brain circuits targeted by drugs, and similarly enhance the efficiency of information processing and thereby relieve symptoms (Figures 6-40 through 6-43).

Experimental animals have epigenetic mechanisms linked not only to spatial memory formation but also to fear conditioning and reward conditioning, models for mood, anxiety, and substance-abuse disorders. Both drugs and psychotherapy can facilitate the formation of new synapses that block memories of fear or reward and provide a potential explanation not only of how psychotherapy can hypothetically change symptoms by altering neuronal circuits, but how combining drugs that facilitate neurotransmission could potentially enhance the efficacy of psychotherapy in changing neuronal circuits, and thus reduce symptoms.

If both psychotropic drugs and psychotherapy converge upon brain circuits, maybe their combination can be harnessed for enhanced efficacy and better outcomes for patients with psychiatric disorders. The question is how to harness the potential of this approach and direct it most effectively to the relief of psychiatric symptoms. What are the techniques, what is the role of the therapist, what training is needed, how can this be standardized and made the most efficient over time with the fastest onset of action, how to measure the neurobiological and symptomatic results of this approach, how to assure that any progress is preserved? We still do not know when to expect greater benefits of psychotherapy alone, medications alone, or their combination, but at least now we have a conceptual basis for using both of them and even for combining them, since the two approaches converge neurobiologically. These and many more questions will form the research agenda for moving this approach forward as a central aspect of clinical therapeutics in psychiatry.

The best psychotherapy candidates to combine with drugs, particularly for the treatment of depression, are cognitive behavioral therapy and interpersonal therapy, which are often conducted by therapists who have read a training manual, been supervised administering it to patients, and who use a 12- to 24-week approach that follows a progression with a beginning, a middle, and an end. The new "trial-based therapy" described by de Oliveira is a version of cognitive psychotherapy that is intuitive, readily adapted by psychiatrists who are not necessarily sophisticated cognitive behavioral therapists, and can even be fun. In trial-based therapy the patient literally puts his psychiatric symptoms and core beliefs on trial. This idea is based on the universal principle portrayed in Franz Kafka's *The Trial* that human beings by their very nature are self-accusatory and this can lead to confusion, anxiety, and existential suffering. In fact, the central character of this novel, Joseph K, was arrested, put on trial, and convicted without ever knowing the crime of which he was accused. De Oliveira's technique is to take this universal truth and fit it into a modern courtroom paradigm. Here, during outpatient psychotherapy, a patient's self-accusations are put on trial as distorted schemas and core beliefs that have been developed about the self by the patient's "inner prosecutor," who convinces the patient that these beliefs are true, and because of this the patient suffers. Trial-based therapy seeks to point out to the patient that his symptoms and suffering are due to core beliefs that can be countered by activating his/her "inner defense attorney" to see things in a more balanced and realistic way and thereby relieve symptoms. One could hypothesize that, when successful, this approach is forming a synapse of the new perspective of the "inner defense attorney" to counter and inhibit the circuit mediating the activation of the first learning, namely the distorted core belief of the "inner prosecutor." Trial-based therapy is only one of the potential psychotherapies to combine with antidepressants for the treatment of major depression and to take us beyond the current plateau of pharmacotherapy. Combining psychotherapy with antidepressants has the potential of making the entire outcome greater than the sum of the parts, or $1 + 1 = 3$, the delightful "bad math" of therapeutic synergy.

How to choose an antidepressant
Evidence-based antidepressant selections

In theory, the best way to select a treatment for depression would be to follow the evidence. Unfortunately, there is little evidence for superiority of one option over another and a good deal of controversy about meta-analyses that compare antidepressants to each other. One general principle upon which most patients and prescribers agree, however, is when to switch versus when to augment. Thus, there is a preference for switching when the first treatment has intolerable side effects or when there is no response whatsoever, but to augment the first treatment with a second treatment when there is a partial response to the first treatment. Other than this guideline, there is little consistent evidence that one treatment option is better than another. All treatments subsequent to the first one seem to have diminishing returns in terms of chances to reach remission (Figure 7-4) or chances to remain in remission (Figure 7-6). Thus, evidence-based algorithms are not able to provide clear guidelines on how to choose an antidepressant, and what to do if an antidepressant does not work.

Symptom-based antidepressant selections

The neurobiologically informed psychopharmacologist may opt for adapting a symptom-based approach to selecting or combining a series of antidepressants (Figures 7-77 through 7-82). This strategy leads to the construction of a portfolio of multiple agents to treat all residual symptoms of unipolar depression until the patient achieves sustained remission.

First, symptoms are constructed into a diagnosis and then deconstructed into a list of specific symptoms that the individual patient is experiencing (Figure 7-77). Next, these symptoms are matched with the brain circuits that hypothetically mediate them (Figure 7-78) and then with the known neuropharmacological regulation of these circuits by neurotransmitters (Figure 7-79). Finally, available treatment options that target these neuropharmacological mechanisms are chosen to eliminate symptoms one by one (Figure 7-79). When symptoms persist, a treatment with a different mechanism is added or switched. No evidence proves that this is a superior approach, but it appeals not only to clinical intuition but also to neurobiological reasoning.

For example, in a patient with the symptoms of "problems concentrating" and "decreased interest" as well as "fatigue," this approach suggests targeting both NE and DA with first-line antidepressants plus augmenting agents that act on these neurotransmitters (Figure 7-79). This can also call for stopping the SSRI if this is partially the cause of these symptoms. On the other hand, for "insomnia," this symptom is hypothetically associated with an entirely different malfunctioning circuit regulated by different neurotransmitters (Figure 7-78); therefore, the treatment for this symptom calls for a different approach, namely the use of hypnotics that act on the GABA system or sedating antidepressants that work to block rather than boost the serotonin or histamine system (Figure 7-79). It is possible that any of these symptoms shown in Figure 7-79 would respond to whatever drug is administered, but this symptom-based approach can tailor the treatment portfolio to each individual patient, possibly finding a faster way of reducing specific symptoms with more tolerable treatment selections for that patient than a purely random approach.

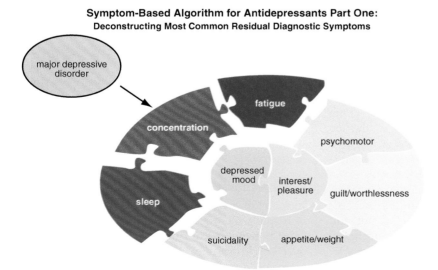

Symptom-Based Algorithm for Antidepressants Part One:
Deconstructing Most Common Residual Diagnostic Symptoms

Figure 7-77. Symptom-based algorithm for antidepressants, part 1. Shown here is the diagnosis of major depressive disorder deconstructed into its symptoms (as defined by formal diagnostic criteria). Of these, sleep disturbances, problems concentrating, and fatigue are the most common residual symptoms.

Symptom-Based Algorithm for Antidepressants Part Two:

Match Most Common Residual Symptoms to Hypothetically Malfunctioning Brain Circuits

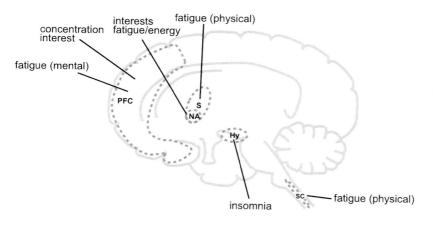

Figure 7-78. Symptom-based algorithm for antidepressants, part 2. In this figure the most common residual symptoms of major depression are linked to hypothetically malfunctioning brain circuits. Insomnia may be linked to the hypothalamus, problems concentrating to the dorsolateral prefrontal cortex (PFC), reduced interest to the PFC and nucleus accumbens (NA), and fatigue to the PFC, striatum (S), NA, and spinal cord (SC).

Symptom-Based Algorithm for Antidepressants Part Three:

Target Regulatory Neurotransmitters With Selected Pharmacological Mechanisms

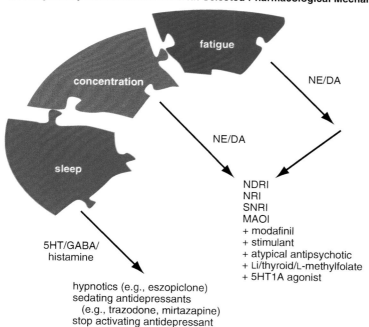

Figure 7-79. Symptom-based algorithm for antidepressants, part 3. Residual symptoms of depression can be linked to the neurotransmitters that regulate them and then, in turn, to pharmacological mechanisms. Fatigue and concentration are regulated in large part by norepinephrine (NE) and dopamine (DA), which are affected by many antidepressants, including norepinephrine–dopamine reuptake inhibitors (NDRIs), selective norepinephrine reuptake inhibitors (NRIs), serotonin–norepinephrine reuptake inhibitors (SNRIs), and monoamine oxidase inhibitors (MAOIs). Augmenting agents that affect NE and/or DA include modafinil, stimulants, atypical antipsychotics, lithium, thyroid hormone, L-methylfolate, and serotonin (5HT) 1A agonists. Sleep disturbance is regulated by 5HT, γ-aminobutyric acid (GABA), and histamine and can be treated with sedative hypnotics, with sedating antidepressants such as trazodone or mirtazapine, or by discontinuing an activating antidepressant.

The symptom-based approach for selecting antidepressants can also be applied to treating common associated symptoms of depression that are not components of the formal diagnostic criteria for depression (Figure 7-80). Five such symptoms are anxiety, pain, excessive daytime sleepiness/hypersomnia/problems with arousal and alertness, sexual dysfunction, and vasomotor symptoms (in women) (Figures 7-80 through 7-82).

The hypothetical pathways for the five additional associated symptoms of depression are shown in Figure 7-81. Sometimes it is said that for a good

Symptom-Based Algorithm for Antidepressants Part Four:
Deconstruct Into Common Non-DSM-IV Residual Symptoms

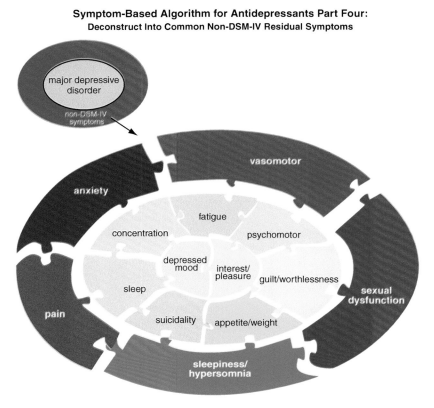

Figure 7-80. **Symptom-based algorithm for antidepressants, part 4.** There are several common symptoms of depression that are nonetheless not part of the formal diagnostic criteria for major depressive disorder. These include painful physical symptoms, excessive daytime sleepiness/hypersomnia with problems of arousal and alertness, anxiety, vasomotor symptoms, and sexual dysfunction.

clinician to get patients with major depression into remission, it requires targeting at least 14 of the 9 symptoms of depression!

Fortunately, psychiatric drug treatments do not respect the formal diagnostic criteria for psychiatric disorders. Treatments that target pharmacological mechanisms in specific brain circuits do so no matter what psychiatric disorder is associated with the symptom linked to that circuit. Thus, symptoms of one psychiatric disorder may be treatable with a proven agent that is known to treat the same symptom in another psychiatric disorder. For example, *anxiety* can be reduced in patients with major depression who do not have a full criterion anxiety disorder with the same serotonin and GABA mechanisms proven to work in anxiety disorders (Figure 7-82). *Sleepiness/ hypersomnia* is a common associated symptom of depression, but frequently not detected because patients who have this problem surprisingly do not often complain about it, while patients with insomnia will much more commonly complain of that if they have that symptom. Problems with the arousal

mechanism in some patients with sleepiness/hypersomnia can also alter alertness and cognitive function, and such patients may respond to the same agents that are effective in sleep disorders, such as agents that can boost DA, NE, and/or histamine (Figure 7-82). We have already discussed *painful physical symptoms* and *vasomotor symptoms* in the section on SNRIs above, neither of which is included in the diagnostic criteria for major depression, both of which are nevertheless commonly associated with depression, and can be treated with SNRIs and other approaches (Figure 7-82). Finally, *sexual dysfunction* can be a complicated problem of many causes, and can range from lack of libido, to problems with arousal of peripheral genitalia, to lack of orgasm/ejaculation. Increasing DA or decreasing 5HT are the usual approaches to this set of problems whether the patient has major depression or not (Figure 7-82).

In summary, the symptom-based algorithm for selecting and combining antidepressants, and for building a portfolio of mechanisms until each diagnostic and associated symptom of depression is abolished, is

Symptom-Based Algorithm for Antidepressants Part Five:
Match Common Non-DSM-IV Residual Symptoms to Hypothetically Malfunctioning Brain Circuits

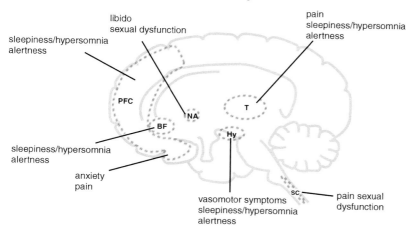

Figure 7-81. Symptom-based algorithm for antidepressants, part 5. In this figure common residual symptoms of major depression that are not part of formal diagnostic criteria are linked to hypothetically malfunctioning brain circuits. Painful physical symptoms are linked to the spinal cord (SC), thalamus (T), and ventral portions of the prefrontal cortex (PFC), while anxiety is associated with the ventral PFC. Vasomotor symptoms are mediated by the hypothalamus (Hy) and sexual dysfunction by the SC and nucleus accumbens (NA). Sleep symptoms that are part of the diagnostic criteria of depression involve mostly insomnia, linked to the hypothalamus; however, shown here are problems with hypersomnia and excessive daytime sleepiness, which may be beyond those symptoms included in the diagnostic criteria and be linked to problems with arousal and alertness and to arousal pathways not only in the hypothalamus but also the thalamus (T), basal forebrain (BF), and prefrontal cortex (PFC).

the modern psychopharmacologist's approach to major depression. This approach follows contemporary notions of neurobiological disease and drug mechanisms, with the goal of treatment being sustained remission.

Choosing an antidepressant for women based on their life cycle

Estrogen levels shift rather dramatically across the female life cycle in relation to various types of reproductive events (Figure 7-83). Such shifts are also linked to the onset or recurrence of major depressive episodes (Figures 7-83). In men, the incidence of depression rises in puberty, and then is essentially constant throughout life, despite a slowly declining testosterone level from age 25 onward (Figure 7-84). By contrast, in women, the incidence of depression in many ways mirrors their changes in estrogen across the life cycle (Figure 7-85). That is, as estrogen levels rise during puberty, the incidence of depression skyrockets in women, falling again after menopause (Figure 7-85). Thus, women have the same frequency of depression as men before puberty and after

menopause. However, during their childbearing years when estrogen is high and cycling, the incidence of depression in women is 2–3 times higher than in men (compare Figures 7-84 and 7-85). Choosing an antidepressant for women in the perimenopause or after the menopause is discussed above in the section on SNRIs.

Depression and its treatment during childbearing years and pregnancy

One of the most controversial and unsettled areas of modern psychopharmacology is the selection of therapeutic interventions for major depressive disorder and prevention of recurrence of depression in women during their childbearing years when they may be pregnant or may become pregnant. What about risks of treatment to the baby? Some antidepressants may pose risks to the fetus, including increased risk for serious congenital malformations if administered during the first trimester and increased risk for other fetal abnormalities and for fetal withdrawal symptoms after birth if administered during the third trimester, and increased risks of

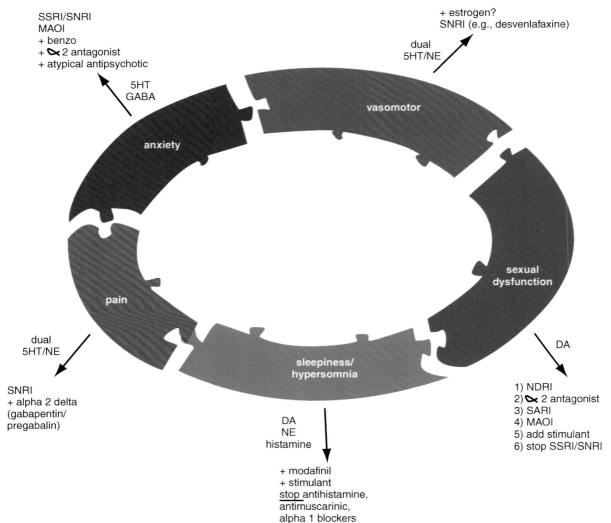

Symptom-Based Algorithm for Antidepressants Part Six:
Target Regulatory Neurotransmitters With Selected Pharmacological Mechanisms

SSRI/SNRI
MAOI
+ benzo
+ ❤ 2 antagonist
+ atypical antipsychotic

5HT
GABA

anxiety

vasomotor

+ estrogen?
SNRI (e.g., desvenlafaxine)

dual
5HT/NE

sexual
dysfunction

pain

DA

dual
5HT/NE

SNRI
+ alpha 2 delta
(gabapentin/
pregabalin)

sleepiness/
hypersomnia

1) NDRI
2) ❤ 2 antagonist
3) SARI
4) MAOI
5) add stimulant
6) stop SSRI/SNRI

DA
NE
histamine

+ modafinil
+ stimulant
stop antihistamine,
antimuscarinic,
alpha 1 blockers

Figure 7-82. Symptom-based algorithm for antidepressants, part 6. Residual symptoms of depression can be linked to the neurotransmitters that regulate them and then, in turn, to pharmacological mechanisms. Painful physical symptoms are mediated by norepinephrine (NE) and to a lesser extent serotonin (5HT) and may be treated with serotonin–norepinephrine reuptake inhibitors (SNRIs) or $\alpha_2\delta$ ligands (pregabalin, gabapentin). Anxiety is related to 5HT and γ-aminobutyric acid (GABA); it can be treated with selective serotonin reuptake inhibitors (SSRIs), SNRIs, or monoamine oxidase inhibitors (MAOIs) as monotherapies, as well as by augmentation with benzodiazepines, α_2 antagonists, or atypical antipsychotics. Vasomotor symptoms may be modulated by NE and 5HT and treated with SNRIs; augmentation with estrogen therapy is also an option. Sexual dysfunction is regulated primarily by dopamine (DA) and may be treated with norepinephrine–dopamine reuptake inhibitors (NDRIs), α_2 antagonists, serotonin 2A antagonist/reuptake inhibitors (SARIs), MAOIs, addition of a stimulant, or by stopping an SSRI or SNRI. Hypersomnia and problems with arousal and alertness are regulated by DA, NE, and histamine and can be treated with activating agents such as modafinil or stimulants, or by stopping sedating agents with antihistamine, antimuscarinic, and/or α_1 blocking properties.

Risk of Depression Across Female Life Cycle

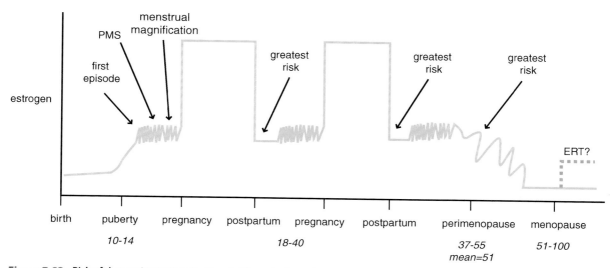

Figure 7-83. Risk of depression across the female life cycle. Several issues of importance in assessing women's vulnerability to the onset and recurrence of depression are illustrated here. These include first onset in puberty and young adulthood, premenstrual syndrome (PMS), and menstrual magnification as harbingers of future episodes or incomplete recovery states from prior episodes of depression. There are two periods of especially high vulnerability for first episodes of depression or for recurrence if a woman has already experienced an episode: namely, the postpartum period and the perimenopausal period. ERT, estrogen replacement therapy.

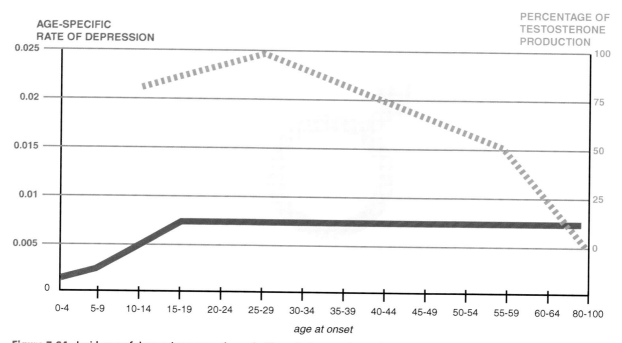

Figure 7-84. Incidence of depression across the male life cycle. In men, the incidence of depression rises in puberty and then is essentially constant throughout life, despite a slowly declining testosterone level from age 25 onward.

AGE-SPECIFIC RATE OF DEPRESSION

PERCENTAGE OF ESTROGEN PRODUCTION

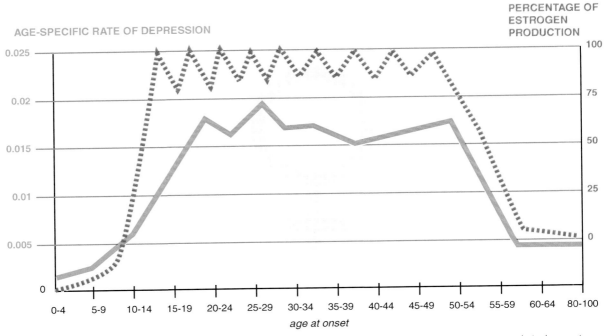

age at onset

Figure 7-85. **Incidence of depression across the female life cycle.** The incidence of depression in women mirrors their changes in estrogen across the life cycle. As estrogen levels rise during puberty, the incidence of depression also rises; it falls again during menopause, when estrogen levels fall. Thus before puberty and after menopause, women have the same frequency of depression as men (Figure 7-84). During their childbearing years, however, when estrogen is high and cycling, the incidence of depression in women is 2–3 times as high as it is in men (Figure 7-84).

prematurity, low birth weight, and possible long-term neurodevelopmental abnormalities if given any time during pregnancy (Table 7-13). At the same time, lack of treatment during pregnancy is not without risks to mother or baby (Table 7-13). For the mother with untreated depression, the risks include relapse or worsening of depression, poor self-care and possible self-harm including resorting to drug abuse of substances even more dangerous than antidepressants (Table 7-13). Not only is there risk of increased suicidality when young mothers are treated with antidepressants, there is also the risk of suicide when seriously depressed mothers of any age are not treated with antidepressants (Table 7-13). There are also numerous risks to the baby if the mother is not treated with antidepressants, including risk of poor prenatal care due to low motivation in the mother, risk of low birth weight and early developmental delay and disruption of maternal–infant bonding in children of women with untreated depression, and even risk of harm to the infant by

seriously depressed mothers in the postpartum period (Table 7-13).

Thus, in terms of treating pregnant patients with antidepressants, it seems that the psychopharmacologist is "damned if you do" and also "damned if you don't" (Table 7-13). Without clear guidelines, clinicians are best advised to assess risks and benefits for both child and mother on a case-by-case basis. For mild cases of depression, psychotherapy and psychosocial support may be sufficient. However, in many cases, the benefits of continuing antidepressant treatment during pregnancy outweigh the risks. L-Methylfolate and folate are actually administered as prenatal vitamins to many women and are deemed safe by most experts. Since patients with unipolar or bipolar depression may be prone to impulsive behavior (especially children and adolescents), it is a good idea for girls and women of childbearing potential who take antidepressants to receive counseling and possibly contraceptives to reduce the risk of unplanned pregnancies and first-trimester exposure of fetuses to antidepressants.

Table 7-13 Risks of antidepressant use or avoidance during pregnancy

Damned if you do

- Congenital cardiac malformations (especially first-trimester paroxetine)
- Newborn persistent pulmonary hypertension (third-trimester SSRIs)
- Neonatal withdrawal syndrome (third-trimester SSRIs)
- Prematurity, low birth weight
- Long-term neurodevelopmental abnormalities
- Increased suicidality of antidepressant use up to age 25
- Medical-legal risks of using antidepressants

Damned if you don't

- Relapse of major depression
- Increased suicidality of antidepressant non-use
- Poor self-care
- Poor motivation for prenatal care
- Disruption of maternal–infant bonding
- Low birth weight, developmental delay in children of women with untreated depression
- Self-harm
- Harm to infant
- Medical-legal risks of not using antidepressants

Depression and its treatment during the postpartum period and while breastfeeding

What about taking antidepressants during the post-partum period, when mothers are lactating and may be nursing? This is a very high-risk period for the onset or recurrence of a major depressive episode in women (Figure 7-83). Should a mother with depression avoid antidepressants in order to prevent risk of exposure of the baby to antidepressants in breast milk? How about a mother with past depression now in remission who is weighing the risk of her own relapse against the risk of exposing the baby to antidepressants in breast milk? In these circumstances there are no firm guidelines that fit all cases, and a risk–benefit ratio must be calculated for each situation, taking into consideration the risk of recurrence to the mother if she does not take antidepressants (given her own personal and family history of mood disorder), and the risk to her bonding to her baby if she does not breastfeed or to her baby if there is exposure to trace amounts of antidepressants in breast milk. Although estrogen replacement therapy (ERT) has been reported to be effective in some

patients with postpartum depression or postpartum psychosis, this is still considered experimental and should be reserved for use if at all only in patients resistant to antidepressants.

Whereas the risk to the infant of exposure to small amounts of antidepressants in breast milk is only now being clarified, it is quite clear that a mother with a prior postpartum depression who neglects to take antidepressants after a subsequent pregnancy has a 67% risk of recurrence if she does not take antidepressants and only one-tenth of that risk of recurrence if she does take antidepressants postpartum. Also, up to 90% of all postpartum psychosis and bipolar episodes occur within the first 4 weeks after delivery. Such high-risk patients will require appropriate treatment of their mood disorder, so the decision here is whether to breastfeed, not whether the mother should be treated.

Choosing an antidepressant on the basis of genetic testing

Genetic testing has the potential of assisting both in diagnosing psychiatric illnesses and in selecting psychotropic drugs. Genotyping is already entering other specialties in medicine, and is currently on the threshold of being introduced into routine mental health practice. In the not-too-distant future, experts foresee that most patients will have their entire genomes entered as part of their permanent electronic medical records. In the meantime, it is already possible to obtain from various laboratories genotyping of numerous genes that may be linked to psychiatric diagnoses and drug responses.

For example, several genetic forms of the cytochrome P450 (CYP) enzyme system can be obtained to predict high or low drug levels of substrate drugs (especially CYP 2D6, 2C19, and 3A4). Combined with therapeutic drug monitoring of actual drug levels, these CYP genotypes can potentially explain side effects and lack of therapeutic effects in some patients.

Treatment responses are not "all or none" phenomena, and genetic markers in psychopharmacology will potentially explain greater or lesser likelihood of response, nonresponse, or side effects, but not tell a clinician what drug to prescribe for a specific individual. More likely, the information will tell whether the patient is "biased" towards responding or not, tolerating or not, and along with past treatment response will help the clinician make a future treatment

Table 7-14 Genetic testing: genes that may help in therapeutic decision making

Gene	Protein	Biological function	Potential therapeutic implications
SLC 6A4 variation	SERT	Serotonin reuptake	Poor response, slow response, poor tolerability to SSRIs/SNRIs
$5HT_{2c}$ variation	$5HT_{2c}$ receptor	Regulates DA & NE release	Poor response, poor tolerability to atypical antipsychotics
DRD_2 variation	D_2 receptor	Mediates positive symptoms of psychosis, movements in Parkinsonism	Poor response, poor tolerability to atypical antipsychotics
COMT Val variation	COMT enzyme	Regulates DA levels in PFC; metabolizes DA and NE	Reduced executive functioning
MTHFR T variation	MTHFR enzyme	Regulates L-methylfolate levels and methylation	Reduced executive functioning, especially with Val COMT (T with Val)

recommendation that has a higher chance of success but is not guaranteed to be effective and tolerated. Some call this process the "weight of the evidence" and others "equipoise," where the genetic information will enrich the prescribing decision, but not necessarily dictate a single compelling choice.

Examples of this are shown in Table 7-14 for several candidate genes that are potentially helpful in weighing various treatment possibilities for patients with treatment-resistant depression. This is a rapidly expanding area of psychopharmacology and will likely impact drug selection dramatically in the next few years.

Should antidepressant combinations be the standard for treating unipolar major depressive disorder?

Given the disappointing number of patients who attain remission from a major depressive episode even after four consecutive treatments (Figure 7-4) and who can maintain that remission over the long run (Figure 7-6), the paradigm of prescribing a sequence of monotherapies each with a single mechanism of therapeutic action for major depression is rapidly changing to one of administering multiple simultaneous pharmacologic mechanisms, often with two or more therapeutic agents. In this respect, the pattern is following that of the treatment of bipolar disorder, which usually requires administration of more than one agent, and of illnesses such as HIV (human immunodeficiency virus) infection as well as tuberculosis. The question in the treatment of depression is not so much whether multiple pharmacologic

mechanisms should be simultaneously administered for patients with treatment-resistant depression, but rather whether multiple mechanisms and/or drugs should be given much earlier in the treatment sequence, or even from the time of initial treatment. Several specific suggestions of antidepressant combinations are shown in Figures 7-86 through 7-88. Many others can be constructed, but these particular combinations or "combos" have enjoyed widespread use even though there is little actual evidence-based data from clinical trials that their combination results in superior efficacy. Nevertheless, these suggestions may be useful for practicing clinicians to use in some patients.

Single-action and multiple-action monotherapies have already been extensively discussed in this chapter, and several combinations of SSRIs/SNRIs with other agents have been mentioned, from atypical antipsychotics (also discussed extensively in Chapter 5), to lithium, buspirone, trazodone, hypnotics, thyroid hormone, L-methylfolate, SAMe, neurostimulation, and psychotherapy. Several additional combos – called "heroic combos" because they have strong anecdotal experience of efficacy in some difficult cases of treatment-resistant depression – are shown in Figures 7-86 through 7-88, including several in which two antidepressants are added together.

Triple-action combo: SSRI/SNRI ± NDRI

If boosting one neurotransmitter is good, and two is better, maybe three boosted neurotransmitters is best (Figure 7-86). Triple-action antidepressant therapy with

Triple-Action Combos

SSRI + NDRI

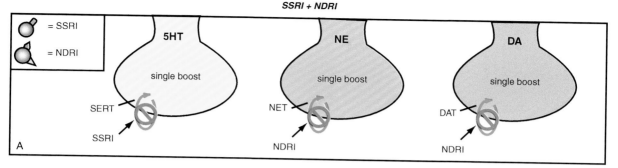

SNRI + NDRI

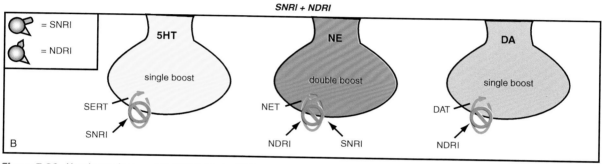

Figure 7-86. Heroic combos, part 1: SSRI/SNRI plus NDRI. A selective serotonin reuptake inhibitor (SSRI) plus a norepinephrine–dopamine reuptake inhibitor (NDRI) leads to a single boost for serotonin (5HT), norepinephrine (NE), and dopamine (DA). A serotonin–norepinephrine reuptake inhibitor (SNRI) plus a norepinephrine–dopamine reuptake inhibitor (NDRI) leads to a single boost for serotonin (5HT), a double boost for norepinephrine (NE), and a single boost for dopamine (DA).

modulation of all three monoamines (5HT, DA, and NE) would be predicted to occur by combining either an SSRI with an NDRI, perhaps the most popular combination in US antidepressant psychopharmacology, or by combining an SNRI with an NDRI, providing even more noradrenergic and dopaminergic action.

California rocket fuel: SNRI plus mirtazapine

This potentially powerful combination utilizes the pharmacologic synergy obtained by adding the enhanced serotonin and norepinephrine release from inhibition of both dual serotonin and norepinephrine reuptake by an SNRI to the disinhibition of both serotonin and norepinephrine release by the α_2 antagonist actions of mirtazapine (Figure 7-87). It is even possible that additional pro-dopaminergic actions result from the combination of norepinephrine reuptake blockade in prefrontal cortex due to SNRI actions with $5HT_{2C}$ actions of mirtazapine

disinhibiting dopamine release. This combination can provide very powerful antidepressant action for some patients with unipolar major depressive episodes. Mirtazapine combinations with various SSRIs and SNRIs have also been studied as potential treatments from the initiation of therapy in major depression.

Arousal combos

The frequent complaints of residual fatigue, loss of energy, motivation, sex drive, and problems concentrating/problems with alertness may be approached by combining either a stimulant or modafinil with an SNRI to recruit triple monoamine action and especially enhancement of dopamine (Figure 7-88). The stimulant lisdexamfetamine, which links the amino acid lysine to the stimulant *d*-amphetamine, and which slows the delivery and potentially reduces the abuse liability of *d*-amphetamine after oral

California Rocket Fuel

SNRI + mirtazapine

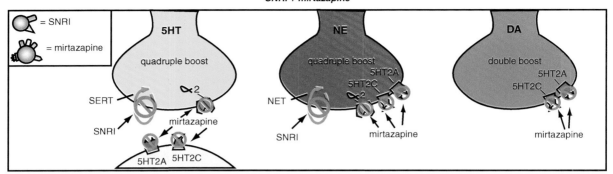

Figure 7-87. Heroic combos, part 2: California rocket fuel. A serotonin–norepinephrine reuptake inhibitor (SNRI) plus mirtazapine is a combination that has a great degree of theoretical synergy: norepinephrine reuptake blockade plus α_2 blockade, serotonin (5HT) reuptake plus $5HT_{2A}$ and $5HT_{2C}$ antagonism, and thus many 5HT actions plus norepinephrine (NE) actions. Specifically, 5HT is quadruple-boosted (with reuptake blockade, α_2 antagonism, $5HT_{2A}$ antagonism, and $5HT_{2C}$ antagonism), NE is quadruple-boosted (with reuptake blockade, α_2 antagonism, $5HT_{2A}$ antagonism, and $5HT_{2C}$ antagonism), and there may even be a double boost of dopamine (with $5HT_{2A}$ and $5HT_{2C}$ antagonism).

Arousal Combos

SNRI + stimulant

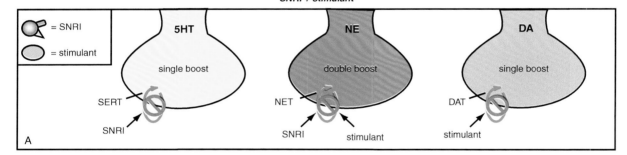

SNRI + modafinil

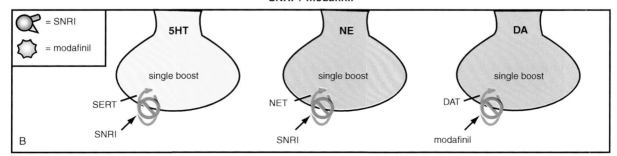

Figure 7-88. Heroic combos, part 3: SNRI plus stimulant or modafinil. A serotonin–norepinephrine reuptake inhibitor (SNRI) plus a stimulant means that serotonin (5HT) and dopamine (DA) are single-boosted and norepinephrine (NE) is double-boosted. With an SNRI in combination with modafinil, serotonin (5HT) and norepinephrine (NE) are single-boosted by the SNRI while dopamine (DA) is single-boosted by modafinil.

administration, is in late-stage clinical testing as an augmenting agent to SSRIs/SNRIs in treatment-resistant depression.

Future treatments for mood disorders

As mentioned in Chapter 6 and illustrated in Figure 6-39B, a number of agents that target stress and the HPA axis are in clinical testing, including *glucocorticoid antagonists, CRF-1 (corticotropin-releasing factor) antagonists* and *vasopressin-1B antagonists*.

Triple reuptake inhibitors (TRIs) or *serotonin–norepinephrine–dopamine reuptake inhibitors* (SNDRIs) are in clinical testing to confirm that if one mechanism is good (i.e., SSRI) and two mechanisms are better (i.e., SNRI), then maybe targeting all three mechanisms of the trimonoamine neurotransmitter system would be the best in terms of efficacy. Several different triple reuptake inhibitors (e.g., amitifidine, GSK-372475, BMS-820836, tasofensine, PRC200-SS, SEP-225289, and others) are in clinical development, some with additional pharmacologic properties (such as LuAA24530 with $5HT_{2C}$, $5HT_3$, $5HT_{2A}$, and α_{1A} antagonist properties), all differing in the amount of blockade of each of the three monoamine transporters SERT, NET, and DAT. It appears that too much dopamine activity can lead to a drug of abuse, and not enough DAT blockade means that the agent is essentially an SNRI. Perhaps the desirable profile is robust inhibition of the serotonin transporter and substantial inhibition of the norepinephrine transporter, like the known SNRIs, plus a little frosting on the cake of 10–25% inhibition of DAT. Further clinical trials will be necessary to clarify whether any of the "triples" will represent an advance over SSRIs or SNRIs in the treatment of depression.

Multimodal agents

It appears that combining multiple modes of monoaminergic action may enhance efficacy for some patients with depression. This can include reuptake blockade (at SERT, DAT, NET) with actions at G-protein receptors (e.g., $5HT_{1A}$, $5HT_{2C}$, $5HT_7$, α_2 receptors) with actions at ion-channel receptors ($5HT_3$ receptors and possibly NMDA receptors). One such agent already discussed is vilazodone (combination of SERT plus $5HT_{1A}$ partial agonist actions) (Figure 7-24). Another multimodal agent

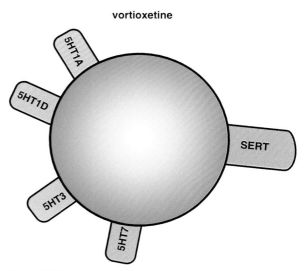

Figure 7-89. Vortioxetine. Vortioxetine is an antidepressant currently in development. It is a serotonin reuptake inhibitor and also has actions at several serotonin receptors, including $5HT_{1A}$ (partial agonist), $5HT_{1B/D}$ (partial agonist), $5HT_3$ (antagonist), and $5HT_7$ (antagonist).

in late-stage clinical development is vortioxetine (LuAA21004) (Figure 7-89). Vortioxetine acts via all three modes with a combination of five pharmacologic actions: reuptake blocking mode (SERT), G-protein receptor mode ($5HT_{1A}$ and $5HT_{1B/D}$ partial agonist, $5HT_7$ antagonist), and ion-channel mode ($5HT_3$ antagonist). In animal models vortioxetine increases the release of five different neurotransmitters: not only triple monoamine action on 5HT, NE, and DA release, but also increases in the release of acetylcholine and histamine. The clinical properties of vortioxetine suggest antidepressant efficacy without sexual dysfunction, and the pharmacologic properties suggest the potential for either pro-cognitive effects, or enhanced antidepressant efficacy compared to agents with fewer modes of action and effects on fewer neurotransmitters. Continued clinical testing will be necessary to see if vortioxetine fulfills its theoretical promise as an antidepressant.

NMDA blockade

One of the most interesting developments in recent years has been the observation that infusions of subanesthetic doses of ketamine can exert an immediate

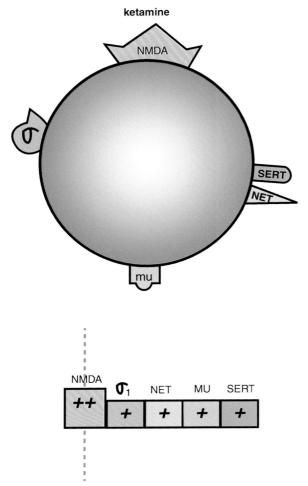

Figure 7-90. Ketamine. Ketamine is being studied for its potential therapeutic utility in depression. Ketamine is an NMDA (*N*-methyl-D-aspartate) receptor antagonist, with additional weak actions at σ_1 receptors, the norepinephrine transporter (NET), μ-opioid receptors, and the serotonin transporter (SERT).

antidepressant effect in patients with treatment-resistant unipolar or bipolar depression, and can immediately reduce suicidal thoughts. Unfortunately, the effects are not sustained for more than a few days, but this has led investigators to search for an oral ketamine-like agent that could have rapid onset and sustained efficacy in treatment-resistant patients.

Ketamine (Figure 7-90) acts as an open channel inhibitor at NMDA glutamate receptors (Figure 7-91), and causes downstream release of glutamate (Figure 7-92). Ketamine's actions at NMDA receptors are not unlike what is hypothesized to occur due to neurodevelopmental abnormalities that occur at NMDA synapses in schizophrenia (Figure 4-29B). This is not surprising, given that ketamine produces a schizophrenia-like syndrome in humans. When infused at subanesthetic doses in the study of depressed patients, ketamine does not induce psychosis, but is thought to produce downstream release in glutamate (Figure 7-92), which stimulates AMPA and mGluR subtypes of glutamate receptors while the NDMA receptors are being blocked by ketamine actions. One hypothesis for why ketamine has antidepressant actions proposes that the stimulation of AMPA receptors first activates the ERK/AKT signal transduction cascade (Figure 7-93A). This next triggers the mTOR (mammalian target of rapamycin) pathway (Figure 7-93A) and that causes the expression of synaptic proteins leading to an increased density of dendritic spines (Figure 7-93B), which can be seen soon after ketamine is administered in animals. Hypothetically, it is this increase in dendritic spines that causes the rapid-onset antidepressant effect.

Thus, investigators are looking for other agents that can trigger the pharmacologic changes that ketamine induces, from blocking NMDA receptors, to stimulating AMPA and various mGlu receptors, to inducing the mTOR pathway and an increase in dendritic spines. One candidate for an "oral ketamine" that acts on NMDA receptors is the cough medicine dextromethorphan (Figure 7-94). Both ketamine and dextromethorphan share actions not only at NMDA receptors, but also at σ receptors, μ-opioid receptors, SERT, and NET, but with different affinities (compare Figures 7-90 and 7-94). Dextromethorphan combined with quinidine (to prevent its metabolism to dextrorphan, which does not penetrate the brain effectively) is available in the US to treat unstable affect known as pseudobulbar affect, and could theoretically act in other disorders of mood and affect – but much more clinical testing is necessary. Many other agents that act on NMDA receptors as potential rapid-acting ketamine-like antidepressants are in early-stage clinical trials.

Site of Action of Ketamine: Binds to Open Channel at PCP Site to Block NMDA Receptor

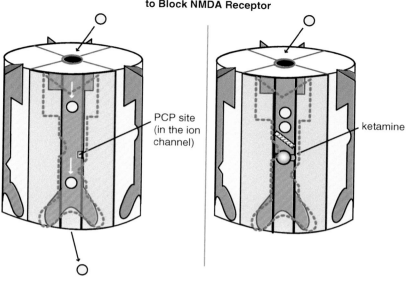

Figure 7-91. Site of action of ketamine. Ketamine binds to the open channel conformation of the *N*-methyl-D-aspartate (NMDA) receptor. Specifically, it binds to a site within the calcium channel of this receptor, which is often termed the PCP site because it is also where phencyclidine (PCP) binds. Blockade of NMDA receptors may prevent the excitatory actions of glutamate, which is postulated to be a therapeutic mechanism for treating depression. In fact, ketamine has demonstrated rapid, short-term antidepressant effects in both animal models and in humans.

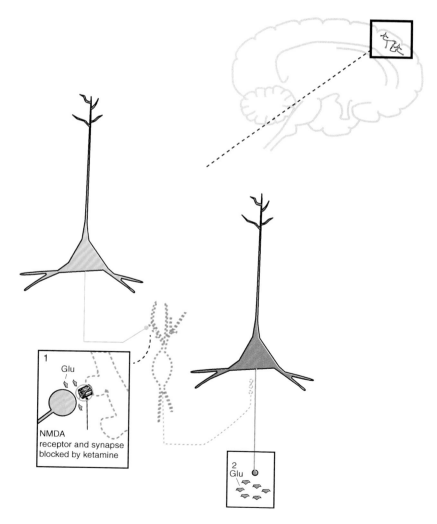

Figure 7-92. Mechanism of action of ketamine. Shown here are two cortical glutamatergic pyramidal neurons and a GABAergic interneuron. (1) If an *N*-methyl-D-aspartate (NMDA) receptor on a GABAergic interneuron is blocked by ketamine, this prevents the excitatory actions of glutamate (Glu) there. Thus, the GABA neuron is inactivated and does not release GABA (indicated by the dotted outline of the neuron). (2) GABA binding at the second cortical glutamatergic pyramidal neuron normally inhibits glutamate release: thus, the absence of GABA there means that the neuron is disinhibited and glutamate release is increased.

131

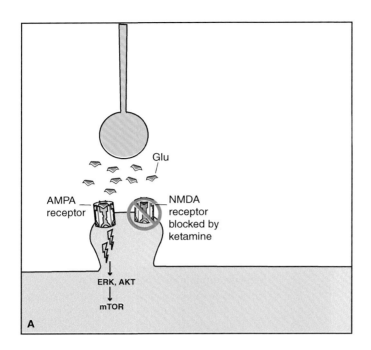

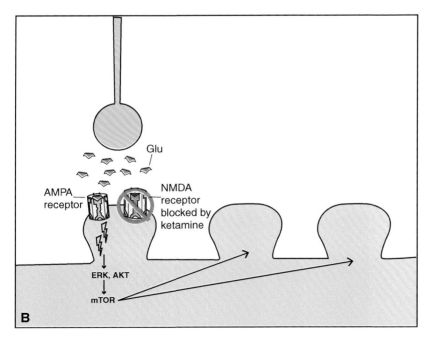

Figure 7-93. Ketamine, AMPA receptors, and mTOR. Glutamate activity heavily modulates synaptic potentiation; this is specifically modulated through NMDA (N-methyl-D-aspartate) and AMPA (α-amino-3-hydroxy-5-methyl-4-isoxazole-propionic acid) receptors. Ketamine is an NMDA receptor antagonist; however, its rapid antidepressant effects may also be related to indirect effects on AMPA receptor signaling and the mammalian target of rapamycin (mTOR) pathway. (A) It may be that blockade of the NMDA receptor leads to rapid activation of AMPA and mTOR signaling pathways. (B) This in turn would lead to rapid AMPA-mediated synaptic potentiation. Traditional antidepressants also cause synaptic potentiation; however, they do so via downstream changes in intracellular signaling. This may therefore explain the difference in onset of antidepressant action between ketamine and traditional antidepressants.

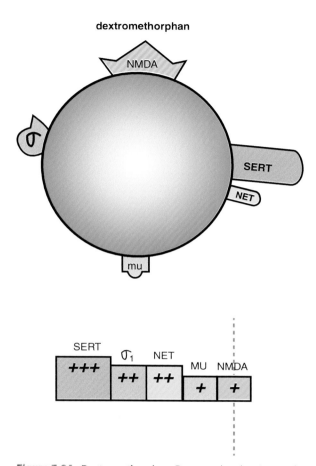

dextromethorphan

Figure 7-94. Dextromethorphan. Dextromethorphan is a weak N-methyl-D-aspartate (NMDA) receptor antagonist, with stronger binding affinity for the serotonin transporter (SERT), σ_1 receptors, and the norepinephrine transporter (NET). It also has some affinity for μ-opioid receptors. Dextromethorphan is approved to treat pseudobulbar affect (in combination with quinidine, which increases its bioavailability) and may have therapeutic utility in depression as well.

Summary

In this chapter, we began with an overview of antidepressant response, remission, relapse, and residual symptoms after treatment with antidepressants. The leading hypothesis for major depression for the past 40 years, namely the monoamine hypothesis, is discussed and critiqued. We have discussed the mechanisms of action of the major antidepressant drugs, including dozens of individual agents working by many unique mechanisms. The acute pharmacological actions of these agents on receptors and enzymes have been described, as well as the major hypothesis – modulation of serotonin, dopamine, and norepinephrine – which attempts to explain how all current antidepressants ultimately work.

Specific antidepressant agents which the reader should now understand include the selective serotonin reuptake inhibitors (SSRIs), serotonin partial agonist/reuptake inhibitors (SPARIs), serotonin–norepinephrine reuptake inhibitors (SNRIs), norepinephrine–dopamine reuptake inhibitors (NDRIs), selective norepinephrine reuptake inhibitors (selective NRIs), α_2 antagonists, serotonin antagonist/reuptake inhibitors (SARIs), MAOIs, tricyclic antidepressants, and melatonergic/monoaminergic antidepressants. We have also covered numerous antidepressant augmenting therapies: atypical antipsychotics, L-methylfolate, SAMe, thyroid, lithium, $5HT_{1A}$ partial agonists, neurostimulation, psychotherapy, stimulants, and the combination of two antidepressants. We have provided some guidance for how to select and combine antidepressants by following a symptom-based algorithm for patients who do not remit on their first antidepressant. We have illustrated some options for combining drugs to treat such patients, and have provided a glimpse into the future by mentioning numerous novel antidepressants on the horizon.

Index